Environmental Health Criteria 209

FLAME RETARDANTS: TRIS(CHLOROPROPYL) PHOSPHATE AND TRIS(2-CHLOROETHYL) PHOSPHATE

Published under the joint sponsorship of the United Nations Environment Programme, the International Labour Organisation, and the World Health Organization, and produced within the framework of the Inter-Organization Programme for the Sound Management of Chemicals.

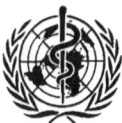

World Health Organization
Geneva, 1998

The **International Programme on Chemical Safety (IPCS)**, established in 1980, is a joint venture of the United Nations Environment Programme (UNEP), the International Labour Organisation (ILO), and the World Health Organization (WHO). The overall objectives of the IPCS are to establish the scientific basis for assessment of the risk to human health and the environment from exposure to chemicals, through international peer review processes, as a prerequisite for the promotion of chemical safety, and to provide technical assistance in strengthening national capacities for the sound management of chemicals.

The **Inter-Organization Programme for the Sound Management of Chemicals (IOMC)** was established in 1995 by UNEP, ILO, the Food and Agriculture Organization of the United Nations, WHO, the United Nations Industrial Development Organization, the United Nations Institute for Training and Research, and the Organisation for Economic Co-operation and Development (Participating Organizations), following recommendations made by the 1992 UN Conference on Environment and Development to strengthen cooperation and increase coordination in the field of chemical safety. The purpose of the IOMC is to promote coordination of the policies and activities pursued by the Participating Organizations, jointly or separately, to achieve the sound management of chemicals in relation to human health and the environment.

WHO Library Cataloguing in Publication Data

Flame retardants : tris(chloropropyl) phosphate and tris(2-chloroethyl) phosphate.

(Environmental health criteria ; 209)

1.Phosphoric acid esters - toxicity 2.Phosphoric acid esters - adverse effects
3.Flame retardants - toxicity   4.Flame retardants - adverse effects
5.Environmental exposure I.International Programme on Chemical Safety
II.Series

ISBN 92 4 157209 4   (NLM Classification: QD 181.P1)
ISSN 0250-863X

PRINTED IN FINLAND
98/12334 – VAMMALA – 5000

CONTENTS

ENVIRONMENTAL HEALTH CRITERIA FOR FLAME RETARDANTS: TRIS(CHLOROPROPYL) PHOSPHATE AND TRIS(2-CHLOROETHYL) PHOSPHATE

NOTE TO READERS OF THE CRITERIA MONOGRAPHS

Every effort has been made to present information in the criteria monographs as accurately as possible without unduly delaying their publication. In the interest of all users of the Environmental Health Criteria monographs, readers are requested to communicate any errors that may have occurred to the Director of the International Programme on Chemical Safety, World Health Organization, Geneva, Switzerland, in order that they may be included in corrigenda.

*   *   *

A detailed data profile and a legal file can be obtained from the International Register of Potentially Toxic Chemicals, Case postale 356, 1219 Châtelaine, Geneva, Switzerland (telephone no. + 41 22 – 9799111, fax no. + 41 22 – 7973460, E-mail irptc@unep.ch).

*   *   *

This publication was made possible by grant number 5 U01 ES02617-15 from the National Institute of Environmental Health Sciences, National Institutes of Health, USA, and by financial support from the European Commission.

Environmental Health Criteria

PREAMBLE

Objectives

In 1973 the WHO Environmental Health Criteria Programme was initiated with the following objectives:

(i) to assess information on the relationship between exposure to environmental pollutants and human health, and to provide guidelines for setting exposure limits;

(ii) to identify new or potential pollutants;

(iii) to identify gaps in knowledge concerning the health effects of pollutants;

(iv) to promote the harmonization of toxicological and epidemiological methods in order to have internationally comparable results.

The first Environmental Health Criteria (EHC) monograph, on mercury, was published in 1976 and since that time an ever-increasing number of assessments of chemicals and of physical effects have been produced. In addition, many EHC monographs have been devoted to evaluating toxicological methodology, e.g., for genetic, neurotoxic, teratogenic and nephrotoxic effects. Other publications have been concerned with epidemiological guidelines, evaluation of short-term tests for carcinogens, biomarkers, effects on the elderly and so forth.

Since its inauguration the EHC Programme has widened its scope, and the importance of environmental effects, in addition to health effects, has been increasingly emphasized in the total evaluation of chemicals.

The original impetus for the Programme came from World Health Assembly resolutions and the recommendations of the 1972 UN Conference on the Human Environment. Subsequently the work became an integral part of the International Programme on Chemical Safety (IPCS), a cooperative programme of UNEP, ILO and WHO. In this manner, with the strong support of the new partners, the importance of occupational health and environmental effects was fully recognized. The EHC monographs have become widely established, used and recognized throughout the world.

The recommendations of the 1992 UN Conference on Environment and Development and the subsequent establishment of the Intergovernmental Forum on Chemical Safety with the priorities for action in the six programme areas of Chapter 19, Agenda 21, all lend further weight to the need for EHC assessments of the risks of chemicals.

Scope

The criteria monographs are intended to provide critical reviews on the effect on human health and the environment of chemicals and of combinations of chemicals and physical and biological agents. As such, they include and review studies that are of direct relevance for the evaluation. However, they do not describe *every* study carried out. Worldwide data are used and are quoted from original studies, not from abstracts or reviews. Both published and unpublished reports are considered and it is incumbent on the authors to assess all the articles cited in the references. Preference is always given to published data. Unpublished data are only used when relevant published data are absent or when they are pivotal to the risk assessment. A detailed policy statement is available that describes the procedures used for unpublished proprietary data so that this information can be used in the evaluation without compromising its confidential nature (WHO (1990) Revised Guidelines for the Preparation of Environmental Health Criteria Monographs. PCS/90.69, Geneva, World Health Organization).

In the evaluation of human health risks, sound human data, whenever available, are preferred to animal data. Animal and *in vitro* studies provide support and are used mainly to supply evidence missing from human studies. It is mandatory that research on human subjects is conducted in full accord with ethical principles, including the provisions of the Helsinki Declaration.

The EHC monographs are intended to assist national and international authorities in making risk assessments and subsequent risk management decisions. They represent a thorough evaluation of risks and are not, in any sense, recommendations for regulation or standard setting. These latter are the exclusive purview of national and regional governments.

Content

The layout of EHC monographs for chemicals is outlined below.

- Summary — a review of the salient facts and the risk evaluation of the chemical
- Identity — physical and chemical properties, analytical methods
- Sources of exposure
- Environmental transport, distribution and transformation
- Environmental levels and human exposure
- Kinetics and metabolism in laboratory animals and humans
- Effects on laboratory mammals and *in vitro* test systems
- Effects on humans
- Effects on other organisms in the laboratory and field
- Evaluation of human health risks and effects on the environment
- Conclusions and recommendations for protection of human health and the environment
- Further research
- Previous evaluations by international bodies, e.g., IARC, JECFA, JMPR

Selection of chemicals

Since the inception of the EHC Programme, the IPCS has organized meetings of scientists to establish lists of priority chemicals for subsequent evaluation. Such meetings have been held in: Ispra, Italy, 1980; Oxford, United Kingdom, 1984; Berlin, Germany, 1987; and North Carolina, USA, 1995. The selection of chemicals has been based on the following criteria: the existence of scientific evidence that the substance presents a hazard to human health and/or the environment; the possible use, persistence, accumulation or degradation of the substance shows that there may be significant human or environmental exposure; the size and nature of populations at risk (both human and other species) and risks for environment; international concern, i.e. the substance is of major interest to several countries; adequate data on the hazards are available.

If an EHC monograph is proposed for a chemical not on the priority list, the IPCS Secretariat consults with the Cooperating Organizations and all the Participating Institutions before embarking on the preparation of the monograph.

Procedures

The order of procedures that result in the publication of an EHC monograph is shown in the flow chart. A designated staff member of IPCS, responsible for the scientific quality of the document, serves as Responsible Officer (RO). The IPCS Editor is responsible for layout and language. The first draft, prepared by consultants or, more usually, staff from an IPCS Participating Institution, is based initially on data provided from the International Register of Potentially Toxic Chemicals, and reference data bases such as Medline and Toxline.

The draft document, when received by the RO, may require an initial review by a small panel of experts to determine its scientific quality and objectivity. Once the RO finds the document acceptable as a first draft, it is distributed, in its unedited form, to well over 150 EHC contact points throughout the world who are asked to comment on its completeness and accuracy and, where necessary, provide additional material. The contact points, usually designated by governments, may be Participating Institutions, IPCS Focal Points, or individual scientists known for their particular expertise. Generally some four months are allowed before the comments are considered by the RO and author(s). A second draft incorporating comments received and approved by the Director, IPCS, is then distributed to Task Group members, who carry out the peer review, at least six weeks before their meeting.

The Task Group members serve as individual scientists, not as representatives of any organization, government or industry. Their function is to evaluate the accuracy, significance and relevance of the information in the document and to assess the health and environmental risks from exposure to the chemical. A summary and recommendations for further research and improved safety aspects are also required. The composition of the Task Group is dictated by the range of expertise required for the subject of the meeting and by the need for a balanced geographical distribution.

EHC PREPARATION FLOW CHART

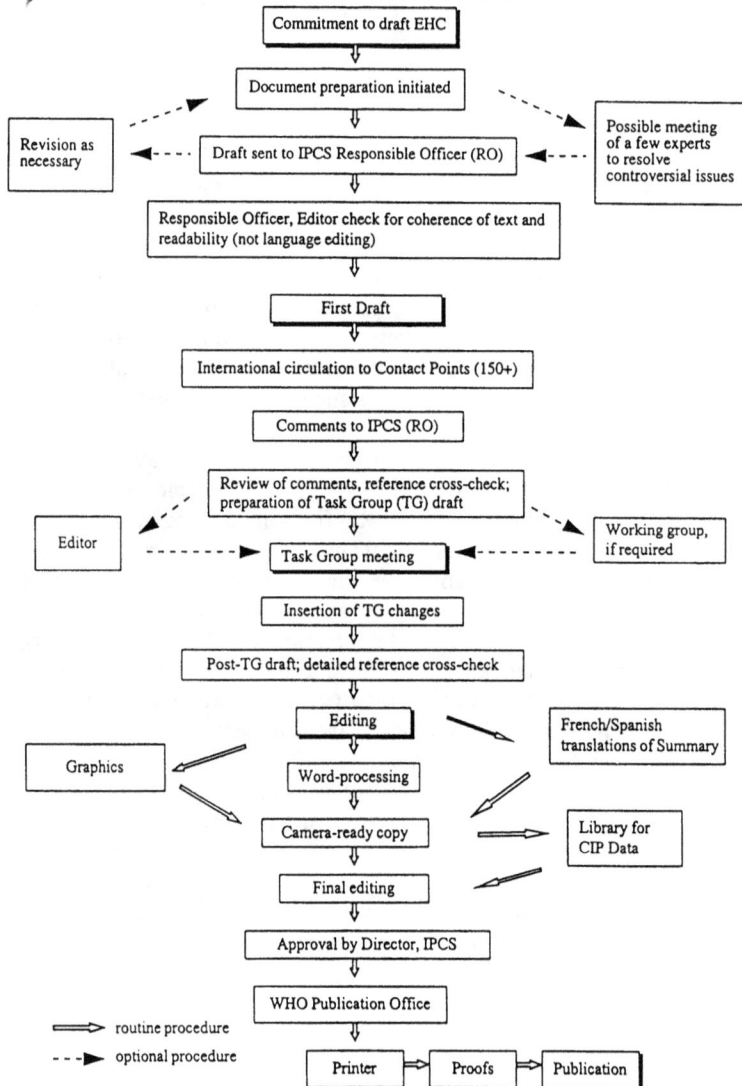

```
                    ┌─────────────────────────────┐
                    │   Commitment to draft EHC   │
                    └─────────────────────────────┘
                                   ⇓
                    ┌─────────────────────────────┐
                    │ Document preparation initiated │
                    └─────────────────────────────┘
                                   ⇓
┌──────────────┐    ┌─────────────────────────────────┐    ┌──────────────────┐
│ Revision as  │◄---│ Draft sent to IPCS Responsible   │◄---│ Possible meeting │
│ necessary    │    │ Officer (RO)                     │    │ of a few experts │
└──────────────┘    └─────────────────────────────────┘    │ to resolve       │
                                   ⇓                        │ controversial    │
                                                            │ issues           │
                                                            └──────────────────┘
        ┌──────────────────────────────────────────────────────────┐
        │ Responsible Officer, Editor check for coherence of text and │
        │ readability (not language editing)                          │
        └──────────────────────────────────────────────────────────┘
                                   ⇓
                        ┌─────────────────┐
                        │   First Draft   │
                        └─────────────────┘
                                   ⇓
        ┌──────────────────────────────────────────────────┐
        │ International circulation to Contact Points (150+) │
        └──────────────────────────────────────────────────┘
                                   ⇓
                    ┌─────────────────────────┐
                    │   Comments to IPCS (RO) │
                    └─────────────────────────┘
                                   ⇓
        ┌──────────────────────────────────────────────────┐
        │ Review of comments, reference cross-check;         │
        │ preparation of Task Group (TG) draft               │
        └──────────────────────────────────────────────────┘
┌──────────┐                       ⇓                        ┌──────────────────┐
│  Editor  │- - - - - ►  ┌────────────────────┐  ◄- - - - - │ Working group,   │
└──────────┘             │ Task Group meeting │             │ if required      │
                         └────────────────────┘             └──────────────────┘
                                   ⇓
                    ┌─────────────────────────┐
                    │ Insertion of TG changes │
                    └─────────────────────────┘
                                   ⇓
        ┌──────────────────────────────────────────────────┐
        │ Post-TG draft; detailed reference cross-check      │
        └──────────────────────────────────────────────────┘
                                   ⇓
                        ┌─────────────────┐              ┌──────────────────────┐
                        │    Editing      │              │ French/Spanish        │
                        └─────────────────┘              │ translations of Summary │
┌──────────────┐                ⇓                        └──────────────────────┘
│  Graphics    │◄─   ┌─────────────────────┐
└──────────────┘     │   Word-processing   │
                     └─────────────────────┘
                                   ⇓
                     ┌─────────────────────┐              ┌──────────────┐
                     │ Camera-ready copy   │─►            │ Library for  │
                     └─────────────────────┘              │ CIP Data     │
                                   ⇓                       └──────────────┘
                        ┌─────────────────┐
                        │  Final editing  │
                        └─────────────────┘
                                   ⇓
                    ┌─────────────────────────┐
                    │ Approval by Director, IPCS │
                    └─────────────────────────┘
                                   ⇓
                    ┌─────────────────────────┐
                    │ WHO Publication Office  │
                    └─────────────────────────┘
                                   ⇓
        ┌─────────┐   ┌─────────┐   ┌──────────────┐
        │ Printer │⇒  │ Proofs  │⇒  │ Publication  │
        └─────────┘   └─────────┘   └──────────────┘
```

⇒ routine procedure

- - -► optional procedure

The three cooperating organizations of the IPCS recognize the important role played by nongovernmental organizations. Representatives from relevant national and international associations may be invited to join the Task Group as observers. While observers may provide a valuable contribution to the process, they can only speak at the invitation of the Chairperson. Observers do not participate in the final evaluation of the chemical; this is the sole responsibility of the Task Group members. When the Task Group considers it to be appropriate, it may meet *in camera*.

All individuals who as authors, consultants or advisers participate in the preparation of the EHC monograph must, in addition to serving in their personal capacity as scientists, inform the RO if at any time a conflict of interest, whether actual or potential, could be perceived in their work. They are required to sign a conflict of interest statement. Such a procedure ensures the transparency and probity of the process.

When the Task Group has completed its review and the RO is satisfied as to the scientific correctness and completeness of the document, it then goes for language editing, reference checking, and preparation of camera-ready copy. After approval by the Director, IPCS, the monograph is submitted to the WHO Office of Publications for printing. At this time a copy of the final draft is sent to the Chairperson and Rapporteur of the Task Group to check for any errors.

It is accepted that the following criteria should initiate the updating of an EHC monograph: new data are available that would substantially change the evaluation; there is public concern for health or environmental effects of the agent because of greater exposure; an appreciable time period has elapsed since the last evaluation.

All Participating Institutions are informed, through the EHC progress report, of the authors and institutions proposed for the drafting of the documents. A comprehensive file of all comments received on drafts of each EHC monograph is maintained and is available on request. The Chairpersons of Task Groups are briefed before each meeting on their role and responsibility in ensuring that these rules are followed.

WHO TASK GROUP ON ENVIRONMENTAL HEALTH CRITERIA FOR FLAME RETARDANTS: TRIS(CHLOROPROPYL) PHOSPHATE AND TRIS(2-CHLOROETHYL) PHOSPHATE

Members

Dr R. Benson, US Environmental Protection Agency, Denver, Colorado, USA (*Rapporteur*)

Mr R. Cary, Health and Safety Executive, Toxicology Unit, Bootle, Merseyside, United Kingdom

Dr S. Dobson, Institute of Terrestrial Ecology, Monks Wood, Huntingdon, Cambridgeshire, United Kingdom

Mr D. Renshaw, Department of Health, London, United Kingdom (*Chairman*)

Dr E. Söderlund, National Institute of Public Health, Department of Environmental Medicine, Oslo, Norway

Dr J. Wagstaff, US Food and Drug Administration, Center for Food Safety and Applied Nutrition, Washington, DC, USA

Observers

Dr R. Henrich, AKZO NOBEL, Dobbs Ferry, New York, USA

Dr P. Martin, Albright and Wilson UK Limited, European Business Services – Product Stewardship, Oldbury, West Midlands, United Kingdom

Mr M. Papez, European Flame Retardants Association (EFRA), c/o European Chemical Industry Council (CEFIC), Brussels, Belgium

Mr D. Thornton, Courtaulds Chemicals, Spondon, Derby, United Kingdom

Secretariat

Dr M. Baril, International Programme on Chemical Safety,
Montreal, Quebec, Canada (*Secretary*)

Dr P.G. Jenkins, International Programme on Chemical Safety,
World Health Organization, Geneva, Switzerland

ENVIRONMENTAL HEALTH CRITERIA FOR FLAME RETARDANTS: TRIS(CHLOROPROPYL) PHOSPHATE AND TRIS(2-CHLOROETHYL) PHOSPHATE

A WHO Task Group on Environmental Health Criteria for Flame Retardants: Tris(chloropropyl) phosphate and Tris(2-chloroethyl) phosphate met at the offices of the Health and Safety Executive (HSE), London, United Kingdom from 9 to 13 March 1998. Drs B. Woodard (HSE) and P. Brantom (British Industrial Biological Research Association) opened the meeting and welcomed the participants on behalf of the organizing institutes. Dr M. Baril, IPCS, welcomed the participants on behalf of Dr M. Mercier, Director of the IPCS and the three cooperating organizations (UNEP/ILO/WHO). The Task Group reviewed and revised the draft monograph and made an evaluation of the risk to human health and the environment from exposure to these flame retardants.

Financial support for this Task Group was provided by the United Kingdom Department of Health as part of its contribution to the IPCS.

The first draft of this monograph was prepared by Dr G. J. van Esch, Bilthoven, the Netherlands. The second draft, prepared by Dr M. Baril, incorporated the comments received following circulation of the first draft to the IPCS contact points for Environmental Health Criteria monographs.

Dr P.G. Jenkins (IPCS Central Unit, Geneva) and Dr M. Baril (IPCS technical adviser, Montreal) were responsible for the overall technical editing and scientific content, respectively.

The efforts of all who helped in the preparation and finalization of the monograph are gratefully acknowledged.

* * *

ABBREVIATIONS

BaP	benzo(a)pyrene
BCF	bioconcentration factor
CA	chromosome aberration
ECD	electron capture detection
FPD	flame photometric detection
GC	gas chromatography
ip	intraperitoneal
LOEC	lowest-observed-effect concentration
LOEL	lowest-observed-effect level
MS	mass spectrometry
NADPH	reduced nicotinamide adenine dinucleotide phosphate
NCI	negative ion chemical ionization
ND	not detectable
NOEC	no-observed-effect concentration
NOEL	no-observed-effect level
NPD	nitrogen phosphorus detection
NTE	neurotoxic esterase
OECD	Organisation for Economic Co-operation and Development
PB	phenobarbital
PCB	polychlorinated biphenyl
SC	subcutaneous
SCE	sister chromatid exchange
TCEP	tris(2-chloroethyl) phosphate
TCPP	tris(1-chloro-2-propyl) phosphate
TDCPP	tris(1,3-dichloro-2-propyl) phosphate
TOCP	tris-*ortho*-cresyl phosphate

TRIS(CHLOROPROPYL) PHOSPHATE

Tris(1-chloro-2-propyl) phosphate
Tris(1,3-dichloro-2-propyl) phosphate

1. SUMMARY

1.1 Tris(1-chloro-2-propyl) phosphate (TCPP)

Tris(1-chloro-2-propyl) phosphate (TCPP) is a colourless liquid used as a flame retardant, mainly in polyurethane foams. It is not volatile. Its solubility in water is 1.6 g/litre, it is soluble in most organic solvents, and it has a log octanol/water partition coefficient of 2.59.

Analysis is by gas chromatography/mass spectrometry (GC/MS). Concentration of TCPP from water prior to analysis can be achieved using XAD resin, followed by extraction with various organic solvents.

TCPP is manufactured from propylene oxide and phosphorus oxychloride. Annual worldwide demand exceeded 40 000 tonnes in 1997.

TCPP is not readily biodegraded in sewage sludge inocula. It is rapidly metabolized in fish.

Traces of TCPP have been detected in industrial and domestic effluents but not in surface waters. It has not been detected in surveys of sediments. Traces of TCPP have been detected in raw peaches, raw pears and fish.

No data are available on the kinetics and metabolism of TCPP in mammals.

TCPP is of low to moderate acute toxicity by the oral (LD_{50} in rats = 1017–4200 mg/kg body weight), dermal (LD_{50} in rats and rabbits is > 5000 mg/kg body weight) and inhalation routes (LC_{50} in rats is > 4.6 mg/litre).

Rabbit eye and skin irritancy studies have indicated that TCPP is either non-irritant or mildly irritant. A skin sensitization study showed that TCPP has no sensitizing properties.

2

The reproductive toxicity, immunotoxicity and carcinogenic potential of TCPP have not been investigated. The results of *in vitro* and *in vivo* mutagenicity studies investigating an appropriate range of end-points indicate that TCPP is not genotoxic.

TCPP has been investigated for potential delayed neurotoxicity in hens. There was no evidence of delayed neurotoxicity when two oral doses (each of 13 230 mg/kg body weight) were given 3 weeks apart.

No studies of the effects of TCPP on humans are available.

Toxicity values for organisms in the environment are available, LC_{50} values ranging from 3.6 to 180 mg/litre. The no-observed-effect concentrations for algae, daphnids and fish are 6, 32 and 9.8 mg/litre, respectively.

1.2 Tris(1,3-dichloro-2-propyl) phosphate (TDCPP)

Tris(1,3-dichloro-2-propyl) phosphate (TDCPP) is a viscous colourless liquid used as a flame retardant in a range of plastic foams, resins and latexes. It is not volatile. Its solubility in water is 0.1 g/litre, it is soluble in most organic solvents, and it has a log octanol/water partition coefficient of 3.8.

Analysis is by GC/MS. Concentration of TDCPP from water prior to analysis can be achieved using XAD resin, followed by extraction with various organic solvents.

TDCPP is manufactured from epichlorohydrin and phosphorus oxychloride. The commercial product is predominantly TDCPP with trace amounts of tris (2,3-dichloropropyl) phosphate. Annual world-wide demand was 8000 tonnes in 1997.

TDCPP is not readily degraded in sewage sludge inocula.

Studies have demonstrated limited degradation of TDCPP in natural waters. It is rapidly metabolized by fish.

Bioconcentration factors are low (3–107). The half-life of elimination in killifish is 1.65 h.

Traces of TDCPP have been detected in sewage effluent, river water, seawater, drinking-water, sediment and in fish. TDCPP has been found in some samples of human adipose tissue.

Kinetic studies in rats using ^{14}C-labelled TDCPP showed the radiolabel to be distributed throughout the body following oral or dermal administration. The major metabolite of TDCPP identified in the urine of rats was bis(1,3-dichloro-2-propyl) phosphate. Elimination of the radiolabel was primarily in faeces and urine, with a small amount in expired air as CO_2.

TDCPP is of low to moderate acute toxicity by the oral route (LD_{50} in rats = 2830 mg/kg body weight) and of low acute toxicity by the dermal route (dermal LD_{50} in rats is > 2000 mg/kg body weight).

In a 3-month study in mice, an exposure of approximately 1800 mg/kg body weight per day caused death within one month. The no-observed-effect level (NOEL) for the study was 15.3 mg/kg body weight per day; the lowest-observed level (LOEL) for increased liver weight was 62 mg/kg body weight per day.

The sensitization potential of TDCPP has not been investigated.

The potential for TDCPP to affect human male reproductive ability is unclear in view of testicular toxicity in rats but a lack of effect on male reproductive performance in rabbits. The possible effect on female reproduction has not been investigated.

A teratology study on rats showed fetotoxicity at an oral dose of 400 mg/kg body weight per day; there was maternal toxicity at doses of 100 and 400 mg/kg body weight per day. No teratogenicity was seen.

Overall, the mutagenicity data show that TDCPP is not genotoxic *in vivo*.

The carcinogenicity of TDCPP has been investigated in a single 2-year feeding study. It was carcinogenic (increased occurrence of liver carcinomas) at all exposure levels that were tested (5–80 mg/kg body weight per day) in both male and female rats. Kidney, testicular and brain tumours were also found. In addition, there were non-neoplastic adverse effects in bone marrow, spleen, testis, liver and kidney. The effects in the kidney and testis occurred at all exposure levels. Only animals in the highest dose and control groups were evaluated for effects in the bone marrow and spleen. It was impossible, therefore, to determine whether there was a dose–response relationship for these effects in these organs.

TDCPP exposure produced some indications of immunotoxicity in mice but only at high doses.

Limited human studies following occupational exposure are available but they add little to the knowledge of the safety aspects of TDCPP.

2. IDENTITY, PHYSICAL AND CHEMICAL PROPERTIES, AND ANALYTICAL METHODS

2.1 Tris(1-chloro-2-propyl) phosphate (TCPP)

2.1.1 Identity

Chemical formula: $C_9H_{18}Cl_3O_4P$

Chemical structure:

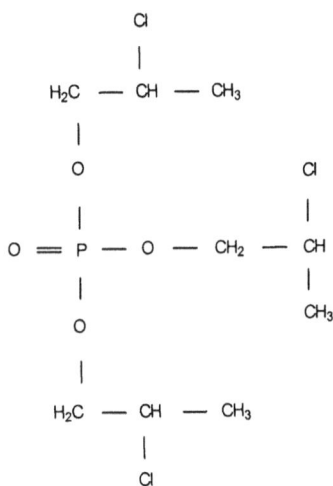

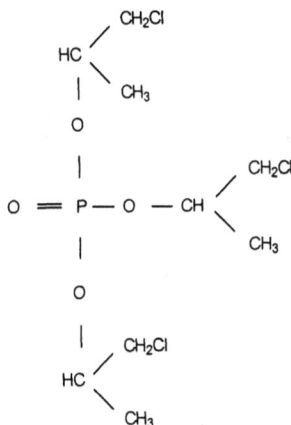

Normal   **ISO**

Relative molecular mass: 327.55

CAS name: tris(2-chloroisopropyl) phosphate

CAS registry number: 13674-84-5

Synonyms: 2-propanol, 1-chlorophosphate (3:1);
                        1-chloro-2-propyl phosphate (1:3);
                        tris(1-chloromethylethyl) phosphate;

tris(2-chloroisopropyl) phosphate;
tris(β-chloropropyl) phosphate;
phosphoric acid, tris(2-chloro-1-methyl
ethyl) ester

Trade names: Fyrol PCF; Amgard TMCP;
Antiblaze 80; Levagard PP; Tolgard
TMCP; TCPP

Common names: TCPP; TMCP; TCIP

2.1.2 *Physical and chemical properties*

Physical state: clear, colourless liquid

Melting point: −42 °C

Boiling point: 235–248 °C

Flash point: 218 °C (Cleveland open cup method)

Vapour pressure: <2 mmHg at 25 °C

Viscosity: 61 cP at 25 °C

Specific gravity: 1.29 at 25 °C

Solubility in water: 1.6 g/litre at 20 °C

Stability: Hydrolyses slowly under alkaline or
acidic conditions

n-Octanol/water partition
coefficient (log P_{ow}):   2.59

References: ECB (1995); Akzo (1995)

2.2   Tris(1,3-dichloro-2-propyl) phosphate (TDCPP)

2.2.1   *Identity*

Chemical formula:	$C_9H_{15}Cl_6O_4P$
Relative molecular mass:	430.91
CAS name:	tris(1,3-dichloroisopropyl) phosphate
CAS registry number:	13674-87-8
Synonyms:	1,3-dichloro-2-propanol phosphate; 2-propanol, 1,3-dichloro-, phosphate; phosphoric acid tris(1,3-dichloro-2-propyl) ester; tris(1-chloromethyl-2-chloroethyl) phosphate; tris(1,3-dichloroisopropyl) phosphate; tris(1,3-dichloro-2-propyl) phosphate; tris [2-chloro-1-(chloromethyl) ethyl] phosphate
Trade names:	CRP; Firemaster T33P; Fyrol FR 2; PF 38; PF 38/3; Apex Flame Proof Emulsion 197 and 212; Antiblaze 195; Amgard; TDCP
Common names:	TDCPP; TDCP

There is some confusion concerning TDCPP isomers. The commercial product has predominantly branched substituent propyl groups in the "iso" orientation joined via the centre carbon. The alternate isomer, i.e. tris(2,3-dichloro-1-propyl) phosphate (CAS registry number 78-43-3), exists only as a trace in the former because of steric hindrance from chlorine substitution on adjacent carbon atoms. Commercial production via reaction of phosphorus oxychloride and epichlorohydrin can, therefore, only produce the major species:

i.e.

```
      Cl              Cl
      |               |
     HC — CH₂ — CH₂
      |
      O              Cl              Cl
      |              |               |
O = P — O — CH — CH₂ — CH₂
      |
      O              Cl
      |              |
     HC — CH₂ — CH₂
      |
      Cl
```

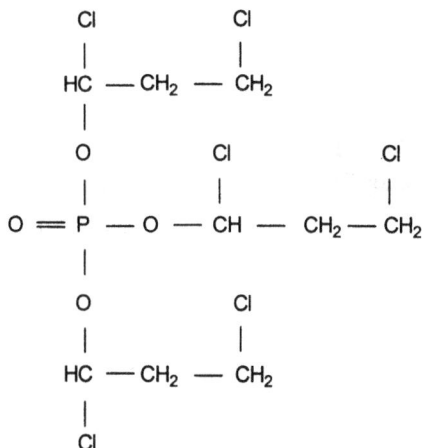

It is therefore assumed that all referenced studies were conducted on commercial samples (CAS registry number 13674-87-4).

2.2.2   *Physical and chemical properties*

Physical state:	viscous liquid
Boiling point:	236–237 °C at 5 mmHg (decomposes at > 200 °C at 4 mmHg)
Specific gravity:	1.52 at 25 °C
Solubility:	0.1 g/litre (30 °C) in water; soluble in most organic solvents
Flash point:	252 °C (Cleveland open cup method)
Stability:	resistant to chlorination in aqueous solution; it has an extremely low rate of hydrolysis and resists attack by bases
Viscosity:	1800 cP (25 °C)

n-Octanol/water partition
coefficient (log P_{ow}):   3.8

Vapour pressure: 0.01 mmHg at 30 °C

References: Hollifield (1979); Sasaki et al. (1981); Windholz (1983); Chemical Information Systems (1988); Ishikawa & Baba (1988); Akzo (1997b)

2.3 Conversion factors

TCPP
> 1 ppm = 0.0746 mg/m^3
> 1 mg/m^3 = 13.39 ppm

TDCPP
> 1 ppm = 0.0567 mg/m^3
> 1 mg/m^3 = 17.62 ppm

2.4 Analytical methods

Gas chromatography and mass spectrometry (GC/MS) with a nitrogen-phosphorus detector (GC/NPD) is used to detect tris(chloropropyl) phosphates in drinking-water and adipose tissue. Water samples are prepared as follows: absorption on a XAD resin cartridge, extraction with methylene chloride or elution with acetone/hexane, drying over anhydrous sodium sulfate and concentration and determination by GC/MS (LeBel et al., 1981; Benoit & LeBel, 1986). LeBel et al. (1987) used large-volume resin sampling cartridges to obtain sufficient organic extracts from water for analysis. Recovery at 10 ng TDCPP/litre fortification was 96.8%.

The limit of determination for tris(chloropropyl) phosphates in human adipose tissue is < 1 ng/g (LeBel & Williams, 1983). The recovery of TDCPP from human adipose tissue fortified with TDCPP was 92.1 to 111.4% in a concentration range of 2.5–25 µg/kg with benzene extraction (LeBel & Williams, 1983).

Gas chromatography with negative chemical ionization mass spectrometry (GC/NCIMS) has been used to identify TDCPP in human blood samples (Sellström & Jansson, 1987).

TDCPP can be analysed in food by GC/NPD (Draft, 1982).

3. SOURCES OF HUMAN AND ENVIRONMENTAL EXPOSURE

3.1 Natural occurrence

Neither TCPP nor TDCPP occur as natural products.

3.2 Anthropogenic sources

3.2.1 Production and processes

TCPP production and use has continued to grow at an average of 4% per year since the mid-1960s when it was first commercialized. Its growth has been a reflection of polyurethane tonnage growth compounded by legislative advances and the fact that TCPP has replaced some other flame retardants, e.g., tris(chloroethyl) phosphate (TCEP).

All commercial TCPP is produced by the reaction of phosphorus oxychloride with propylene oxide followed by purification.

All commercial TDCPP is produced by reaction of phosphorus oxychloride with epichlorohydrin.

In 1997, global TCPP demand reached over 40 000 tonnes per year; global TDCPP demand was estimated at 8000 tonnes per year and growing.

3.2.2 Release in the environment

The environmental fate of TCPP is unknown; entry into and transport through the aquatic media, however, appear to be the most likely sources of contamination. TCPP fire retardants could potentially reach the environment from waste streams generated: (a) in manufacturing plants; (b) where they are added to fabrics and plastics; and (c) from the final product during its use, disposal or recycling. Their transport to the environment could also occur by atmospheric emissions, by leaching or with the movement of treated fabrics or plastic products (US EPA, 1976).

Ahrens et al. (1979) determined the rate of release of TDCPP as a function of the number of launderings of children's polyester sleepwear. They observed that about 37% of the flame retardant was lost after 20 washings, most of which was lost by the tenth wash. Pre-polymers containing polyethyleneimine with TDCPP impart flame retardancy to cotton fabrics but do not withstand persistent laundering (Bertoniere & Rowland, 1977).

TDCPP may undergo thermal oxidative degradation in air at 370 °C. The major chlorinated C3 species (97% volatiles) are 1,3-dichloropropene and 1,2,3-trichloropropane and acrolein. Hydrochloric acid is also produced.

3.2.3   Uses

3.2.3.1   TCPP

The vast majority of TCPP is used in rigid polyurethane foams. It is also used in flexible polyurethane foams for furniture and its upholstery, principally in the United Kingdom and Ireland.

TCPP is added at various points in the polyurethane supply chain: to final foam producers; to "system houses" who pre-blend and formulate ready-made systems; and to base polyol producers who may use it to reduce polyol viscosity/mobility.

The use in rigid polyurethane foams may be further sub-divided into blocks and spray systems for building insulation and for refrigerator casings. Very small use of TCPP also exists in textile back-coating formulations and in certain coatings.

3.2.3.2   TDCPP

TDCPP is added as a flame retardant to: (a) polyurethane foam (both rigid and flexible); (b) other plastics and resins; and (c) acrylic latexes for back coating and binding of non-woven fabrics (Weil, 1980; US EPA, 1988).

Incorporation of TDCPP into polyurea coatings for application to wool has produced flame-resistant, machine-washable and shrink-resistant material (Fincher et al., 1973).

TDCPP was formerly used as a flame retardant for children's and infant's clothing.

4. ENVIRONMENTAL TRANSPORT, DISTRIBUTION AND TRANSFORMATION

4.1 Transport and distribution between media

No data are available regarding transport and distribution of TCPP or TDCPP between different media.

4.2 Transformation

4.2.1 Abiotic

TCPP hydrolyses slowly under both acidic and alkaline conditions (Akzo, 1997a).

4.2.2 Biotic

TCPP is not readily biodegradable in sewage sludge inocula. Following inoculation at 20 mg/litre in a MITI test, 14% was degraded in 28 days (MITI, 1992). After inoculation at 100 mg/litre in a test under OECD Guideline 3OI C, there was no degradation within 28 days (Bayer AG, 1990, unpublished data). Using Amgard TMCP, TCPP was assessed for inherent biodegradability under OECD Guideline 302C. Calculated degradation (from oxygen uptake) was 21% after 28 days (SafePharm, 1996a). In the same test, Amgard TDCP (TDCPP), showed no degradation within 28 days (SafePharm, 1996b).

4.2.3 Degradation

Hattori et al. (1981) studied the degradation of TDCPP in environmental water during 1979–1980. Using the molybdenum blue colorimetric method, the increase of phosphate ions was analysed in Oh River and Neya River water and seawater from Osaka Bay. According to measurements made at 7 and 14 days, the degradation was 12.5 and 18.5%, respectively, when 20 mg TDCPP/litre was added to water from the Oh River, 0 and 5.4%, respectively, when 1 mg/litre was added to water from the Neya River, 0 and 22%

respectively in seawater from Osaka Bay (Tomagashima), and 0% in seawater from Osaka Bay (Senboku).

The percentage degradation of TDCPP in water in the presence of killifish (*Orzyias latipes*) or goldfish (*Carassius auratus*) was monitored by Sasaki et al. (1981). Initial concentration and fish numbers per unit volume were not reported. More than 90% of the TDCPP degradation with killifish, and approximately 70% with goldfish, occurred within 100 h; the half-lives being 31 h for killifish and 42 h for goldfish.

4.2.4   Bioaccumulation

Bioaccumulation of TDCPP was studied in both static and continuous-flow tests using killifish (*Oryzias latipes*). In static tests, bioconcentration factors (BCFs) ranged from 47 to 107 following exposure to TDCPP at 0.3–1.2 mg/litre for 96 h. In continuous-flow systems, BCFs ranged from 31 to 59 following exposure to 0.04–0.4 mg/litre over 3 to 32 days. The half-life of elimination was 1.65 h following transfer to clean water after exposure in the continuous-flow system (Sasaki et al., 1982). Static BCFs for goldfish (*Carassius auratus*) ranged from 3 to 5 for TDCPP (Sasaki et al., 1981).

5. ENVIRONMENTAL LEVELS AND HUMAN EXPOSURE

5.1 Environmental levels

5.1.1 Air

TCPP and TDCPP concentrations of 0.0053 and 0.0047 $\mu g/m^3$, respectively, were measured in the ambient air of Kitakyushu, Japan, in 1983 (Haraguchi et al., 1985).

5.1.2 Water

In 1975 and 1978 more than 100 samples of river water were analysed in Japan for the presence of TDCPP. In 1975 0/100 and in 1978 0/114 samples contained the substance. The limit of determination in 1975 was 0.02–0.25 and in 1978 it was 0.001–0.5 $\mu g/litre$ (Environmental Agency Japan, 1983, 1987).

In a survey conducted in 1980, 25 samples of river water and seawater were collected near Kitakyushu City, Japan, and analysed for TDCPP. All samples contained this phosphate at concentrations of 0.023–0.136 $\mu g/litre$ (limit of determination, 0.01 $\mu g/litre$) (Ishikawa et al., 1985a).

Twenty-four samples of water were collected and analysed for the presence of TDCPP in Japan in 1984. None of the samples contained either TDCPP (limit of determination 0.25–1 $\mu g/litre$) or TCPP (limit of determination 0.05–1 $\mu g/litre$) (Environmental Agency Japan, 1987; personal communication from the Japanese Ministry of Health and Welfare to the IPCS, July 1993).

TDCPP has been identified in raw river water and drinking-water extracted from Japanese rivers (Takahashi & Morita, 1988). A study of river water samples collected at Isojima in the Yodo river basin in 1984 led to the conclusion that urban run-off was not a source of river water pollution in that area (Fukushima et al., 1986). Fukushima et al. (1992) determined the trend of TCPP and TDCPP levels in the basin from 1976 to 1990. There was a peak in the polluted area of TDCPP in 1987 where the concentration reached 0.9 µg/litre and one in a less polluted area in 1988 where it was 0.6 µg/litre.

Industrial and domestic effluents in Kitakyushu, Japan, contained detectable levels of TDCPP (limit of determination, 0.03 µg/litre). The concentration ranged from not detectable (ND) to 0.1 µg/litre at 3 food factories, ND to 0.6 µg/litre at 7 chemical factories, ND to 0.29 µg/litre at 5 steel factories, ND to 0.59 µg/litre at 6 other industrial sites and ND to 0.18 µg/litre at 3 metal processing plants, 0.28 to 1.4 µg/litre in 5 sewage treatment plant effluents (influents 0.33 to 1.6 µg/litre) and ND to 0.56 µg/litre in 5 domestic effluents. It was concluded by the authors that the water pollution in the area was due to a combination of pollution sources of low concentrations (Ishikawa et al., 1985b). TCPP was detected at 0.06 µg/litre only in one of the "other industrial sites" and was not detected in other industrial effluents. TCPP was found at only one of the sewage treatment plants (at 0.98 µg/litre in the influent and 0.32 µg/litre in the effluent).

TDCPP was detected at concentrations ranging from trace to 0.22 µg/litre in water from water treatment plants in Japan (Takahashi & Morita, 1988).

In 1979 a survey of drinking-water from treatment plants throughout Canada was carried out. Samples were taken approximately 3 months apart in August/September and again in November/December. TDCPP was found at levels ranging from 0.0003 to 0.023 µg/litre in the drinking-water supply of 15 Canadian cities. It was not detected in drinking-water from 14 other cities (Williams & LeBel, 1981).

The concentration of TDCPP in drinking-water samples (one sample at each station) collected in 1980 from 12 Canadian Great Lakes municipalities ranged up to 0.0157 µg/litre during January and from 0.0001 to 0.0046 µg/litre during August (Williams et al., 1982). Drinking-water samples (two samples of each station) collected from six Eastern Ontario water treatment plants, in the period June–October 1978, contained 0.0002 to 0.0018 µg/litre (LeBel et al., 1981).

In a survey of organic effluent pollutants from three Swedish waste water treatment plants, Paxéus (1996) found TDCPP at concentrations of < 0.5 to 3 µg/litre.

5.1.3 Sediment

In 1975, 100 samples and, in 1978, 114 samples of sediment were analysed for the presence of TDCPP in Japan. No TDCPP was found (limit of determination in 1975 was 0.002–0.05 and, in 1978, 0.0001–0.06 mg/kg) (Environmental Agency Japan, 1983, 1987).

In a survey in 1980, four out of six samples of sediment collected from a river and the sea near Kitakyushu City, Japan, contained TDCPP at concentrations of 9–17 µg/kg (limit of determination, 5 µg/kg) (Ishikawa et al., 1985a).

Twenty-four samples of sediment were collected and analysed for the presence of TDCPP and TCPP in Japan in 1984. None of the samples contained TDCPP (limit of determination, 0.03–0.06 mg/kg) or TCPP (limit of determination, 0.011–0.05 mg/kg) (Environmental Agency Japan, 1987; personal communication from the Japanese Ministry of Health and Welfare to the IPCS, July 1993).

5.1.4 Biota

In 1975 and in 1978 samples of Japanese fish were analysed for the presence of TDCPP. In 1975, 7/94 samples contained TDCPP at concentrations of 0.015–0.025 mg/kg and in 1978 0/93 samples contained TDCPP (limit of determination, 0.001–0.03 mg/kg) (Environmental Agency Japan, 1983, 1987).

5.1.5 Food

In a market-basket survey of 234 food items conducted over a 10-year period between 1982 and 1991, TCPP was found 3 times. Residues found in raw peach and raw pear were 0.009 mg/kg (limits of detection unspecified) (Kan-Do Office and Pesticides Team, 1995).

5.2   General population exposure

5.2.1   Adipose tissue

In a series of studies (LeBel & Williams, 1983, 1986; LeBel et al., 1989), TDCPP was detected in human adipose tissue. In initial studies, concentrations ranged from not detectable (< 0.001 µg/kg) to 257 µg/kg. In later studies, samples from 4 out of 6 cities showed no detectable TDCPP, whilst in the other two concentrations ranged up to 32 µg/kg.

5.2.2   Biological fluids

Using NCI mass spectrometry with a limit of detection of 0.01 µg, Hudec et al. (1981) found TDCPP in the seminal fluid of 34 out of 123 student donors. The TDCPP concentrations ranged from 5 to 50 µg/litre.

6. KINETICS AND METABOLISM IN LABORATORY ANIMALS

6.1 TCPP

No data are available on the kinetics or metabolism of TCPP.

6.2 TDCPP

The only data available derive from studies in rats.

Groups of 2–8 male Sprague-Dawley rats received an unstated amount of ^{14}C-TDCPP by intravenous injection (Lynn et al., 1981). The position of the radiolabel was not specified. Urine, faeces and expired air were collected for 24-h periods over 5 days; bile and plasma samples were collected over 24 h only. Total radiolabel and tissue concentrations of TDCPP were assessed in most major organs at 5 min, 30 min, 8 h, 24 h and 5 days after injection. The major metabolite isolated from urine, faeces and bile was 1,3-dichloro-2-propyl phosphate (BDCP); in addition 1,3-dichloro-2-propanol and a dimethyl derivative of BDCP were identified in urine. There was also substantial elimination of ^{14}CO$_2$ via exhaled air. The tissue distribution studies indicated distribution of the parent compound and the major metabolite (1,3-dichloro-2-propyl phosphate) throughout the body. On completion of 5 days collection, approximately 96% of the administered radiolabelled material had been recovered in the urine, faeces or exhaled air.

Similar results were reported following dermal application of 0.9 mg/kg and oral administrations of up to 22 mg/kg (Nomeir et al., 1981; Minegishi et al., 1988).

Following the intraperitoneal administration of ^{14}C-TDCPP to male Sprague-Dawley rats, urine collected over 24 h contained a major metabolite, bis(1,3-dichloro-2-propyl) phosphate (BDCPP) (Lynn et al. 1981). In rats receiving intravenous injection, 54% of the radiolabel was excreted in the urine after 5 days; 62% of the urinary label was BDCPP (Lynn et al., 1980,1981).

Nomeir et al. (1981) studied the metabolism of ^{14}C-TDCPP in rats. Labelled TDCPP was distributed rapidly throughout the body following either oral or dermal administration or intravenous injection. Elimination of TDCPP was primarily in the bile, faeces and urine, but some was expired as CO_2. About 80% of the dose was eliminated within 24 h, but traces of radioactivity were found in most tissues 10 days following exposure.

In a similar study, Minegishi et al. (1988), using male Wistar rats, showed, after 168 h of an oral administration of 21.5 mg/kg in olive oil, a recovery of 43.2% in the urine, 39.2% in the faeces and 16.2% in the expired air.

Six hours after intravenous administration of ^{14}C-TDCPP (40.7 mg/kg) to CD-1 mice, binding of TDCPP-derived radioactivity was detected in isolated RNA, DNA and protein from liver, kidney and muscle. The maximum levels in RNA, DNA and protein were 28, 8.3 and 57 nmoles/kg, respectively (Morales & Matthews, 1980).

TDCPP was rapidly metabolized *in vitro* by an NADPH-dependent microsomal mixed-function oxidase system and glutathione S-transferases from rat liver to BDCPP, 1,3-dichloro-2-propanol, 3-chloro-1,2-propanediol, and one metabolite which was probably a glutathione conjugate (Nomeir et al., 1981; Sasaki et al., 1984).

7. EFFECTS ON LABORATORY MAMMALS AND *IN VITRO* TEST SYSTEMS

7.1 Single exposure

7.1.1 TCPP

Acute oral LD_{50} values for TCPP in rat have been reported in a series of studies, as presented in Table 1, and range between 931 and 4200 mg/kg body weight for males and 707 and 2500 mg/kg body weight for females.

LC_{50} values for inhalation exposure to TCPP administered as an aerosol to rats are given in Table 2.

Dermal LD_{50} values for the rat and for the rabbit are above 2000 mg/kg body weight (Gordon, 1980; Smithey, 1981c; Cuthbert, 1989f).

7.1.2 TDCPP

Slc/ddY mice (10 male, 10 female per group) were given a single oral intubation of TDCPP in olive oil and were observed for 14 days. There were 7 dose groups and a control group for males and 6 dose groups and a control group for females. The dose range was 2210–3500 mg/kg for males and 1890–2780 mg/kg for females. Clinical signs included ataxia, hyperactivity and convulsion (incidence not reported). LD_{50} values for male and female mice were 2670 mg/kg (range 2520–2830) and 2250 mg/kg (range 2120–2390 mg/kg), respectively (Kamata et al., 1989).

In two different studies using male and female Sprague-Dawley rats, Cuthbert (1989a,b) investigated the oral and dermal LD_{50} of TDCPP. In the oral study, clinical signs noted 1–5 days after dosing included hypokinesia, piloerection, soiled coats, ataxia, chromoda-cryorrhoea, rhinorrhoea and salivation. In the dermal study, no death occurred and no clinical signs were noted 24 h after administration. In both cases the LD_{50} was evaluated as greater than 2000 mg/kg.

Table 1. Oral LD$_{50}$ values for TCPP in rats

Strain[a]	LD$_{50}$ (mg/kg body weight)		Clinical signs	Reference
	Male	Female		
Sprague-Dawley	4200	2800	"depression", tremors, lacrimation, salivation, convulsion	Stauffer, 1979
Sprague-Dawley	2710	–	"depression" and tremors at dosage > 1000 mg/kg	Stauffer, 1972
Sprague-Dawley	2000	1260	"depression" and intermittent muscle spasm at 464 mg/kg; salivation ataxia and spasmodic jumping at high dose	Stauffer, 1970
Sprague-Dawley	931	–	"depression" hunched posture, decreased respiratory rate, increased salivation, laboured respiration	Safepharm (undated/a)
Sprague-Dawley	1310	–	hunched posture, decreased respiratory rate, signs of lethargy, ataxia, laboured respiration	Safepharm (undated/c)
Sprague-Dawley	–	980	ataxia, hunched posture, decreased respiratory rate, lethargy, laboured respiration	Safepharm (undated/d)
Sprague-Dawley	–	1548	ataxia, hunched posture, lethargy, piloerection, decreased respiratory rate, laboured respiration	Safepharm (undated/e)
NS	–	1011	piloerection, hunched posture, waddling gait, lethargy, respiratory distress, increased salivation, clonic convulsions	Huntingdon Life Sciences, 1997b
NS	–	707	hunched posture, waddling gait, lethargy, respiratory distress, increased salivation	Huntingdon Life Sciences, 1997a

Table 1 (contd).

NS	1546	1017	increased or reduced activity; oral, nasal, perional and ocular discharge, hunching, rough coat, aggression, diarrhoea, anorexia and sporadic twisting	Mehsl, 1980
NS	1824	1101	reduced activity, oral/nasal discharge, convulsion, emaciation, prostration	Anon, 1981a
NS	1750	1150	—	Bayer AG, 1990 (unpublished data)
NS	1419[b]			Stauffer, 1978 (Report No. T6539)
NS	>2000[b,c]		After 1–3 days, reduced activity, piloerection and ataxia	Cuthbert, 1989d

[a] NS = not specified
[b] Separate values for males and females not given
[c] 10 animals (5 of each sex)

Table 2. LC$_{50}$ values for TCPP administered as aerosol to rats

Duration (h)	LC$_{50}$ (mg/litre)	Remarks[a]	Reference
1	> 17.8	10 animals (5 of each sex), whole body exposure; clinical signs: decreased activity, partially closed eyes, swollen eye lids, lacrimation	Mehlman & Smart, 1981
4	> 4.6	clinical signs: mild lethargy and matted fur	Stauffer, 1979
4	> 7.9	10 animals (5 of each sex)	Anderson, 1990a
4	approximately 5 (female) > 5 (male)	whole body exposure (one exposure level only; 0/5 male; 3/5 female); clinical signs: decreased activity, increased salivation	Mehlman & Singer, 1981

[a] There were no deaths in the first three studies but three females out of five died in the study of Mehlman & Singer (1981)

When Anderson (1990b) administered a TDCPP-containing aerosol to groups of 5 male and female Sprague-Dawley rats, the LC_{50} was greater than 5220 mg/m^3.

7.2   Short-term exposure

7.2.1   TCPP

Groups of rats fed ad libitum for 14 days at levels of 4200, 6600, 10 600 and 16 600 mg/kg diet presented minimal evidence of toxicity. No treatment-related changes were seen in haematology, clinical chemistry or cholinesterases activity. Increased relative and absolute liver weights were reported without concomitant histopathological change (Stauffer, 1980).

7.2.2   TDCPP

No histological effects were observed in the liver, kidneys or gonads of rats given daily doses of 250 mg/kg per day for 10 days (Ulsamer et al., 1980).

7.3   Long-term exposure

7.3.1   TCPP

No data on TCPP are available.

7.3.2   TDCPP

Slc/ddY mice (12 male, 12 female per group) were administered diets containing 0, 100, 400, 1300, 4200 or 13 300 mg/kg diet for 3 months. The daily intake of TDCPP reported by the authors was 0, 13, 47, 171, 576 or 1792 mg/kg body weight per day for males and 0, 15, 62, 214, 598 or 1973 mg/kg body weight per day for females. The animals in the highest exposure groups showed emaciation, rough hair and tremor (incidence not reported) and all animals died within one month. Haemoglobin concentration was decreased in males and females by 13% and 11%, respectively, in the group treated with 4200 mg/kg diet.

There was a progressive increase in serum alkaline phosphatase and serum alanine aminotransferase activities with increasing exposure, but the change was not statistically significant after 3 months. There was also an increase in relative liver weight in males (statistically significant in the 1300 and 4200 mg/kg groups where the increases were 32% and 51%, respectively) and females (statistically significant in the 400, 1300 and 4200 mg/kg groups, where the increases were 16%, 29% and 51%, respectively). There was also an increase in relative kidney weight in males (statistically significant in the 4200 mg/kg group where the increase was 39%) and females (statistically significant in the 1300 and 4200 mg/kg groups where the increases were 34% and 40%, respectively). A slight necrosis was reported in the liver of two females of the 4200 mg/kg group. In this study the NOEL for the increase in relative liver weight in males was 47 mg/kg body weight per day and in females 15 mg/kg body weight per day; the LOEL in males was 171 mg/kg body weight per day and in females 62 mg/kg body weight per day (Kamata et al., 1989).

7.4 Skin and eye irritation or sensitization

7.4.1 TCPP

7.4.1.1 Skin irritation

TCPP was investigated in New Zealand white rabbits for dermal irritation. Two reports classified TCPP as mild or slightly irritant to rabbit skin (Cuthbert, 1989e; Safepharm, 1979c).

In a study conducted under OECD Test Guideline 404, 0.5 ml TCPP was applied to the skin of three New Zealand white rabbits under a semi-occlusive dressing for 4 h (Liggett & McRae, 1991a). Slight erythema (grade 1) was noted in one animal on day 1 only. Thereafter, there were no signs of skin irritation.

In two different studies, 0.5 ml of TCPP was applied to two test sites, one abraded and one intact skin of the back of six New Zealand white rabbits under an occlusive binder for 24 h. Using the technique of Draize test, sites were scored for irritancy at 24 and 72 h after application. In both case the test material was classified as not irritant (Smithey, 1980b, 1981b).

7.4.1.2   Eye irritation

In a study conducted under OECD Test Guideline 405, 0.1 ml TCPP was instilled into one eye of each of three New Zealand white rabbits (Liggett & McRae, 1991b). Slight conjunctival redness (grade 1) was seen in each animal on day 1 only. Thereafter, there were no signs of eye irritation.

Three older studies conducted under different guidelines using albinos or New Zealand white rabbits reported no signs of eye irritation (Safepharm, 1979b; Smithey, 1980a, 1981a). In a limited study, Cuthbert & Jackson (1990b) reported that TCPP was slightly irritant, but the effect was quickly reversible in New Zealand white rabbits.

7.4.1.3   Sensitization

TCPP was examined using the Magnuson and Kligman method for possible contact sensitization potential in guinea-pigs. TCPP produced no skin sensitization(Safepharm, 1979a).

7.4.2   TDCPP

7.4.2.1   Skin irritation

The acute dermal irritation potential of TDCPP was investigated in three New Zealand white rabbits. Well defined (score 2) erythema was recorded in 2 animals 1 h after patch removal. The third animal showed very slight erythema at 1 h. By 48 h all treated sites were normal. TDCPP was classified as irritant to rabbit skin (Cuthbert, 1989c).

7.4.2.2   Eye irritation

New Zealand white rabbits were used to evaluate the eye irritation potential of TDCPP. Slight conjunctival redness and slight discharge were noted 1 h after instillation. By 24 h after instillation, all treated eyes were normal. It was concluded that TDCPP was slightly irritant to the rabbit eye (Cuthbert & Jackson, 1990a).

7.4.2.3   Sensitization

No data on the skin sensitization potential of TCPP are available.

7.5   Reproductive toxicity, embryotoxicity and teratogenicity

7.5.1   TCPP

No studies concerning the possible reproductive toxicity, embryotoxicity or teratogenicity of TCPP have been reported.

7.5.2   TDCPP

Female Wistar rats (15–24 per group) were given 25, 50, 100, 200 or 400 mg/kg body weight by oral intubation on days 7 to 15 of gestation. In the 400 mg/kg group, there was severe maternal toxicity; maternal body weight gain and food consumption were markedly suppressed and 11 out of 15 dams died. Clinical signs in dams at 400 mg/kg included piloerection, salivation and haematuria. Fetal death was markedly increased at 400 mg/kg. In the 200 mg/kg group there was a statistically significant increase in relative kidney weight (15% increase) in dams. No effects on dams were seen at lower exposures. There was no evidence of an increased number of fetal deaths, of abnormal fetal development, or of malformation at an exposure of 200 mg/kg or less. In this study the NOEL and LOEL for maternal toxicity were 100 mg/kg and 200 mg/kg body weight per day, respectively, and the NOEL and LOEL for fetotoxicity were 200 mg/kg and 400 mg/kg body weight per day, respectively (Tanaka et al., 1981).

In a fertility study, male rabbits were given oral gavage TDCPP doses of 2, 20 or 200 mg/kg body weight per day for 12 weeks. The treatment did not affect mating behaviour, fertility, sperm quality or sperm quantity. Kidney and liver weight were increased at 200 mg/kg body weight per day, but it was reported that no histopathological lesions were seen in kidneys, liver, pituitaries, testes or epididymes (Wilczynski et al., 1983).

7.6 Mutagenicity and related end-points

7.6.1 TCPP

There was no clear evidence from a battery of assays for mutagenicity and related effects to suggest that TCPP was genotoxic (Tables 3 and 4).

TCPP produced no gene mutations in strains TA1535, TA1537, TA1538, TA97, TA98 and TA100 in any of six Salmonella/microsome plate assays and one *Escherichia coli* (Stauffer, 1978c; Nakamura et al., 1979; Anon, 1980; Zeiger et al., 1992; Mehlman et al., 1980; Parmar, 1977; Kouri & Parmar, 1977) nor in a yeast gene mutation assay (Stauffer, 1978c) in either the presence or absence of metabolic activation. One mouse lymphoma assay gave equivocal results (Anon, 1981b), but a second mouse lymphoma assay was negative in the presence and absence of metabolic activation (Stauffer, 1978a). An *in vitro* assay for unscheduled DNA synthesis (UDS) in a primary culture of rat hepatocytes gave a negative result (Bayer, 1991, Report No. 20393), whereas the results of *in vitro* UDS assays in WI-38 cells (Stauffer, 1978b) were equivocal in the presence and absence of metabolic activation. Two out of three cell transformation assays in BALB/3T3 cells gave negative results in the absence of metabolic activation (Stauffer, 1978b, 1980, Report No. T10182), whereas the third was equivocal (Stauffer, 1978, Report No. T6357).

TCPP caused no chromosomal damage in bone marrow in three *in vivo* cytogenetic assays using oral or subcutaneous administration to rats (Stauffer, 1978, Report No. T6539) and intraperitoneal administration to mice (Bayer, 1991, Report No. 20029).

7.6.2 TDCPP

TDCPP has been tested for mutagenic effects *in vitro* and *in vivo* (Tables 5 and 6).

Table 3. Mutagenicity and related end-points for TCPP *in vitro*

Test system	Concentration	Activation +S9	Activation -S9	Result[a]	Reference
Bacterial gene mutation assays					
Salmonella typhimurium TA100, TA1535	0.3–10 μmol/plate	+	+	–	Nakamura et al., 1979
Salmonella typhimurium TA97, TA98, TA100, TA1535, TA1537	3.3–1000 μg/plate	+	+	–	Zeiger et al., 1992
Salmonella typhimurium TA98, TA100, TA1535, TA1537, TA1538	0.001–5 μl/plate	+	+	–	Stauffer, 1978c
Salmonella typhimurium TA98, TA100, TA1535, TA1537, TA1538	0.03–1 μl/plate	+	+	–	Anon, 1980
Salmonella typhimurium TA98, TA100, TA1535, TA1537, TA1538	0.03–0.33 μl/plate	+	+	–	Mehlman et al., 1980
Salmonella typhimurium TA98, TA100, TA1535, TA1537, TA1538	1–50 μl/plate	+	+	–	Parmar, 1977
Escherichia coli Pol A +, Pol A –	2–20 μl/plate	+	+	–	Kouri & Parmar, 1977
Yeast gene mutation assay					
Saccharomyces cerevisiae	0.001–5 μl/plate	+	+	–	Stauffer, 1978c
L5178Y TK+/–	0.08–0.48 μl/ml	+	+	–	Stauffer, 1978c
L5178Y TK+/–	0.006–0.028 μl/ml	+	+	±	Anon, 1981b

Table 3 (contd).

Unscheduled DNA synthesis					
Human diploid WI-38 cells	0.1–5 µl/ml	+	+	±	Stauffer, 1978b
Human diploid WI-38 cells	0.1–100 µl/ml	+	–	±	Stauffer, 1978b
Rat liver primary cells	12.5–200 µg/ml	+	–	–	Bayer, 1991 (Report No. 20393)
Cell transformation assays					
BALB/3T3 cells	0.00125–0.02 µl/ml	–	+	±	Stauffer, 1978 (Report No. T6357)
BALB/3T3 cells	0.00125–0.02 µl/ml	–	+	–	Stauffer, 1978b
BALB/3T3 cells	0.00015–3 µl/ml	–	+	–	Stauffer, 1980 (Report No. T10182)

[a] ± = equivocal result

Table 4. *In vivo* mutagenicity assays for TCPP

Species	Route of administration	Dose	Result	Reference
Cytogenetic assays				
Rat	oral	0.011, 0.04 and 0.11 ml/kg body weight	no chromosomal aberrations	Stauffer, 1978 (Report No. T6539)
Rat	subcutaneous	0.011, 0.04 and 0.11 ml/kg body weight on 5 consecutive days	no chromosomal aberrations	Stauffer, 1978 (Report No. T6539)
Mouse	intraperitoneal	350 mg/kg body weight	"no clastogenic effects"	Bayer, 1991 (Report No. 20029)

Table 5. Mutagenicity and related end-points for TDCPP *in vitro*

Test system	Concentration	Result	Reference
Bacterial tests			
S. typhimurium TA100, TA1535, G46	10–200 µg/plate	+	Brusick et al., 1980
S. typhimurium TA97, TA98, TA100, TA1535, TA1537	10 to 10 000 µg/plate	+	Mortelmans et al., 1986
S. typhimurium TA100	50–1000 µg/plate	+	Søderlund et al., 1985
S. typhimurium TA100	50–250 µg/plate	+	Gold et al., 1978
Mouse lymphoma assay			
L5178Y cells	up to 0.07 µl/ml	–	Brusick et al., 1980
SCE assay			
L5178Y cells	0.005–0.07 µl/ml	?	Brusick et al., 1980
Chromosomal aberration assays			
L5178Y cells	0.01–0.1 µl/ml	+	Brusick et al., 1980
CHL cells	?	+	Kawachi et al., 1980; Ishidate et al., 1981
Human fibroblasts	?	–	Kawachi et al., 1980; Ishidate et al., 1981
Cell transformation			
BALB/3T3 cells	up to 0.312 µl/ml	–	Brusick et al., 1980

Table 6. *In vivo* mutagenicity of TDCPP

Test system[a]	Dose	Result	Reference
Insect assay			
SLRL mutations in Drosophila	2.5 and 25% in feed	–	Brusick & Jagannath, 1977; Brusick et al., 1980
Mammalian bone marrow assays			
SCE & CA in CD1 mice	0.05–0.5 ml/kg body weight	–	Brusick et al., 1980
Micronuclei in mice	2000 mg/kg body weight	–	Thomas & Collier, 1985

[a] SLRL = sex-linked recessive lethal
SCE = sister-chromatid exchange
CA = chromosome aberration

TDCPP has been investigated several times in bacterial gene mutation studies using the *Salmonella*/microsome mutation test. Mortelmans et al. (1986) reported the findings of four tests performed in three different laboratories which tested TDCPP using strains TA100, TA1535, TA98, TA97 (2 labs) and TA1537 (2 labs) in the presence and absence of metabolic activation by S9 from Aroclor 1254 activated livers of rats and hamsters. There was no evidence of mutagenicity in the absence of S9, but all three laboratories obtained some positive results in the presence of S9. Positives were reported in at least some of the laboratories for strains TA97, TA100 and TA1535 with both hamster and rat S9. All three laboratories reported positive findings in TA100. Two other studies (Gold et al., 1978; Søderlund et al., 1985) also found a mutagenic response in TA100 in the presence of metabolic activation. Brusick et al. (1980) found no mutagenicity in strains TA1535 or G46 in the presence or absence of S9, but obtained different results in TA100 depending upon the source of the S9 used in the assay: mutagenic activity was seen when they used S9 from rat liver activated with Aroclor 1254 or phenobarbital but not with S9 from human liver or from mouse liver activated with Aroclor 1254 or phenobarbital. Taken as a whole, the results of bacterial tests show TDCPP to have mutagenic potential.

No mutagenic activity was noted in strains TA98, TA100, TA1535 or TA1537 when they were incubated with untreated or beta-glucuronidase-treated urine from TDCPP-treated mice (Brusick et al., 1980). The CD1 mice had been given oral doses of 0.05, 0.17 or 0.5 ml/kg body weight per day, and urine was collected on the fourth day of treatment. It was unclear from the report of the study whether or not the urine samples had been tested for mutagenicity in the presence of any metabolizing system.

TDCPP did not induce gene mutations in the mouse lymphoma assay either in the absence or presence of various exogenous metabolic systems (S9 from rat or mouse liver induced with either Aroclor 1254 or phenobarbital) when tested up to a concentration causing a 50% reduction in cell growth (Brusick et al., 1980).

TDCPP was also tested for *in vitro* chromosome effects, i.e. chromosomal aberrations (CA) and sister chromatid exchanges (SCE), using mouse lymphoma (L5178Y) cells at concentrations up to those causing a 50% reduction in growth rate (Brusick et al., 1980). Tests were performed in the absence and presence of various exogenous metabolic systems (S9 from mouse liver induced with either Aroclor 1254 or phenobarbital). The results for SCEs were equivocal, whereas those for CAs showed increased numbers of chromosomal aberrations (excluding gaps) with both metabolic activation systems. Induction of SCEs was reported in a separate study by Gold et al., 1978. Incomplete reports of *in vitro* cytogenetic studies claimed that TDCPP caused chromosomal aberrations in CHL cells but not in human fibroblasts (Kawachi et al., 1980; Ishidate et al., 1981).

TDCPP did not induce primary DNA damage as measured indirectly as unscheduled DNA synthesis in a primary culture of rat hepatocytes (Williams et al., 1989). *In vivo* covalent binding studies in CD1 mice have revealed that TDCPP and/or its metabolites can bind to cellular DNA from the liver and kidney (Morales & Matthews, 1980). Section 6.2 includes other details of this study.

TDCPP did not induce sex-linked recessive lethal mutations in *Drosophila melanogaster* (Brusick et al., 1980).

TDCPP did not induce SCEs or CAs in bone marrow cells of CD1 mice (sex not reported) following either a single oral gavage dose of 0.05, 0.17 or 0.5 ml TDCPP/kg body weight (using bone marrow harvest times of 6, 24 and 48 h post-dosing) or 5 consecutive daily oral exposures at the same dose levels with a harvest time of 6 h after the last dose (Brusick et al., 1980).

TDCPP did not induce micronuclei in polychromatic erythrocytes in the bone marrow of either sex of mice (strain not reported) that had been given a single dose of 2000 mg TDCPP/kg body weight by an unspecified route of administration (Thomas & Collier, 1985). The ratio of normochromatic erythrocytes to polychromatic erythrocytes was not elevated at any of the sampling times (24, 48 and 72 h post-dosing), but, as there was systemic toxicity seen in the treated mice, the TDCPP must have entered the blood circulation and thus the bone marrow cells must have been exposed to TDCPP and/or its metabolites.

TDCPP did not induce morphological cell transformations in BALB/3T3 cells in two independent tests in the absence of any metabolic activation (Brusick et al., 1980).

7.7 Carcinogenicity

7.7.1 TCPP

No data on the carcinogenic potential of TCPP are available.

7.7.2 TDCPP

Groups of 50 male and 50 female Sprague-Dawley rats received approximately 0, 5, 20 and 80 mg TDCPP/kg per day by dietary administration for 2 years (Aulette & Hogan, 1981). An additional 10 animals per group were killed after 1 year for interim investigations. Examinations included body weight gain and food consumption, haematology, clinical chemistry, urinalysis, ophthalmoscopy, organ weights and extensive macroscopic and microscopic investigations.

Increased mortality was reported in males at 80 mg/kg per day. Reduced body weight gain was noted in males and females at 80 mg/kg per day (approximately 20% lower than control), although food consumption was unaffected. Ophthalmoscopy revealed sacculations on the retinal arterioles in one male at 20 mg/kg per day and four males and four females at 80 mg/kg per day at 80 or 104 weeks. Red blood cell values were reduced amongst males and females at 80 mg/kg per day. In addition, there was a slight decrease in plasma cholinesterase activity in females at 80 mg/kg per day, although erythrocyte cholinesterase was unaffected.

Increased liver, kidney and thyroid weights were reported at 12 and 24 months at the highest dose in both males and females. Microscopic pathology changes were observed in liver, kidneys, testes (and associated tissues), bone marrow, spleen and parathyroids. In the liver, a slight increase in the occurrence of local hepatocellular alterations was noted in males and females at 80 mg/kg per day (males, 29/46 compared to 20/45 in controls; females, 35/50 compared to 15/49 in controls). In addition, there was a slight increase in the incidence of dilated sinusoids in the liver at this exposure level (males, 12/46 compared to 4/55; females, 18/50 compared to 7/49). In the kidneys, an increased occurrence of hyperplasia in the convoluted tubules was observed in all groups of treated males and females (males, 2/45, 10/49, 28/48, 24/46; females 0/49, 1/48, 3/48, 22/50). In addition, there was an increase in the occurrence of chronic nephropathy in males and females at 80 mg/kg per day (males, 39/46 compared to 25/45; females, 25/50 compared to 7/49). In the seminiferous tubules there was a slight increase in the occurrence of germinal epithelial atrophy and oligospermia (30/43, 29/48, 42/47, 44/45); eosinophilic material in the tubular lumen (2/43, 4/48, 12/47, 11/45); sperm stasis (5/43, 5/45, 11/47, 14/45); periarteritis nodosa (5/43, 10/48, 19/47, 14/45). Seminal vesicle atrophy and decreased secretory products were reported in all treated groups. In the epididymides males given 80 mg/kg per day had an increased incidence of oligospermia and degenerated seminal products.

An increased incidence of bone marrow erythroid/myeloid hyperplasia was recorded in males and females at 80 mg/kg (males, 21/42 compared to 12/40 in controls; females, 18/44 compared to 13/41). However, no samples were taken from other treated groups.

An increased incidence of spleen erythroid/myeloid metaplasia was seen in males and females at 80 mg/kg per day (males, 10/45 compared to 12/45 in controls; females, 33/50 compared to 30/49). Again there were insufficient tissue samples taken from other treatment groups to draw firm conclusions about the dose–response relationship. Similarly, there was an increased occurrence of parathyroid hyperplasia in males and females at 80 mg/kg per day (males, 12/31 compared to 1/21; females, 9/25 compared to 6/26). Insufficient samples were taken from other treated groups to determine the dose–response relationship.

Neoplastic changes were observed in the liver, kidneys, testes, brain, thyroid and adrenals. In liver, the occurrence of benign neoplastic nodules was 2/45, 7/48, 1/48, 13/46 in males and 1/49, 1/47, 4/46, 8/50 in females; the incidence of carcinoma was 1/45, 2/48, 3/48, 7/46 in males and 0/49, 2/47, 2/46, 4/50 in females. In the kidneys the incidence of renal cortical tumours (benign and/or malignant) was

1/45, 3/49, 9/48, 32/46 in males and 0/49, 1/48, 8/48, 49/50 in females. The incidence of benign testicular interstitial tumours was 7/43, 8/48, 23/47 and 36/45. A slight increase in the incidence of brain astro-cytomas was observed in males receiving 80 mg/kg per day (4/46 compared to 0/44 in controls) and a single oligodendroglioma was observed amongst males and females given 80 mg/kg per day.

The occurrence of thyroid adenomas was increased amongst females at 80 mg/kg per day (5/49 compared to 1/42 in controls). In addition, a slight increase in the occurrence of parafollicular cell adenomas was noted in males and females at 80 mg/kg per day (males, 3/41 compared to 0/40; females, 4/49 compared to 2/42). The occurrence of adrenal cortical adenomas was increased only in females at 80 mg/kg per day (19/49 compared to 8/48 in controls).

It was concluded that TDCPP is carcinogenic at all exposure levels that were tested in both sexes of rats based on the increased occurrence of liver carcinomas. Kidney, testicular and brain tumours were also found. In addition, there were non-neoplastic adverse effects in bone marrow, spleen, testis, liver and kidney. Effects in the kidney and testis occurred at all exposure levels. Only the animals in the highest dose and control groups were evaluated for effects in the bone marrow and spleen. It was impossible, therefore, to determine the dose–response relationship for these effects.

7.8 Other studies

7.8.1 Immunotoxicity

7.8.1.1 TCPP

No data on the immunotoxic potential of TCPP are available.

7.8.1.2 TDCPP

The effects of TDCPP on immunological functions and host susceptibility to infectious agents were examined following exposure in adult mice. Groups of 7–10 B6C3F$_1$ mice received 0, 0.25, 2.5 or 25 mg/kg per day by subcutaneous injection for 4 days. Immunological tests included bone marrow cellularity and colony formation, lymphoproliferative responses to mitogens, delayed hypersensitivity and serum IgG, IgM, and IgA concentrations. Other end-points examined included clinical signs of toxicity, haematology, clinical chemistry, body weight, and the weight of thymus, spleen and liver. There were no clinical signs of toxicity, no significant effects on body weight, organ weight, and no abnormal histopathology.

TDCPP treatment induced minimal changes in immune functions and host susceptibility only at the highest dose tested. This was indicated by decreased ($P < 0.05$) lymphoproliferative responses to mitogens and increased tumour takes following tumour cell challenge, where there was an increase ($P < 0.05$) in the number of animals with tumours (8/10 versus 5/10 in control) but no change in the latency period (Luster et al., 1981).

7.8.2 Neurotoxicity

7.8.2.1 TCPP

The neurotoxic potential of TCPP in adult white Leghorn hens was evaluated by Sprague et al. (1981). A group of 18 hens received an initial oral dose of 13.23 g TCPP/kg body weight followed by the same treatment 3 weeks later. The animals were sacrificed 3 weeks after the second dose. Loss of body weight, transient reduction in food consumption and one death were reported for the treated animals. Egg production ceased shortly after the first dose and there was severe loss of feathers. No behavioural or histological evidence for delayed neurotoxicity was seen.

7.8.2.2 TDCPP

Chickens exposed orally to TDCPP at doses of 0.6, 1.2, 2.4 or 4.8 g/kg body weight per day for 5 days exhibited leg and wing weakness at doses of 1.2 g/kg or more and 100% mortality at 4.8 g/kg body weight, while lower dose levels caused leg and wing weakness (Ulsamer et al., 1980).

White Leghorn hens, 12 months old, were orally exposed to 420 mg TDCPP/kg body weight per day for five consecutive days as specified in the procedure outlined in Navy MIL-H-19457B (SHIPS) protocol. After 21 days of observation there were no signs of neurotoxicity, whereas TOCP, used as positive control, induced inability to walk, hypertension, ataxia and prostration (Bullock & Kamienski, 1972).

8. EFFECTS ON HUMANS

8.1 TCPP

No data concerning the effects of TCPP on humans are available.

8.2 TDCPP

A retrospective cohort study examined mortality in 289 workers employed in the manufacture of TDCPP. The cohort included all male workers employed for 3 months or more in a manufacturing plant in the USA during 1956–1977. The subjects were followed up until 1980. Overall mortality in the subjects was 75% of the normal expected for the male population in the USA. Three cases of cancer of the lung were identified (0.8 cases expected), but all three decedents were moderate to heavy smokers. Air samples were not taken at the time of exposure but breathing zone samples were taken from other area/job classifications in 1981 and all contained less than 0.4 $\mu g/m^3$ (7 ppb) of TDCPP. The slight increase in the number of people with lung cancer was not statistically significant and its association with TDCPP exposure remains unclear due to the small size of this study, the absence of evidence of exposure to TDCPP, the effect of possible mixed exposure to other chemicals and other confounding factors including smoking history (Stauffer, 1983b).

During 1981 workers at a TDCPP manufacturing plant in the USA had their health assessed in physical examinations. The health reports of 93 potentially exposed workers from the factory were compared with the health reports of 31 non-exposed workers who were matched for age, alcohol consumption and smoking habits. The two groups of workers were comparable with regard to chest X-ray results. Exposed workers had a 2-fold increase in the prevalence of "abnormal" electrocardiograms, but fewer exposed workers had a history of heart disease. There were no significant differences in any of the clinical chemistry parameters investigated. The prevalence of minor respiratory disease was slightly increased in exposed workers. The results of the study did not reveal any significantly increased morbidity in workers exposed to TDCPP (Stauffer, 1983a).

9. EFFECTS ON OTHER ORGANISMS IN THE LABORATORY AND FIELD

9.1 Microorganisms

The LC_{50} for bacteria from sewage sludge was reported to be > 10 000 mg/litre for TDCPP (Akzo, 1997b). No data were identified for TCPP.

9.2 Aquatic organisms

9.2.1 Algae

The EC_{50} for growth has been reported to be 47 mg TCPP/litre for the green alga *Selenastrum capricornutum* (Akzo, 1997c). The corresponding EC_{50} in the same alga for TDCPP was 12 mg/litre (Akzo, 1997b). Exposure of the alga *Scenedesmus subspicatus* to TDCPP (Amgard TDCP) at 10 mg/litre for 72 h had no effect on growth or biomass (SafePharm, 1994).

9.2.2 Invertebrates

The 48-h LC_{50} for *Daphnia* was reported to be 131 mg/litre (measured concentration corresponding to 209 mg/litre nominal concentration) for TCPP as Antiblaze 80 under static conditions (Mobil, 1985a). A lower-observed-effect concentration (LOEC) (based on nominal concentrations) of 33.5 mg/litre was determined on the basis of behavioural observations.

A 21-day reproduction test using *Daphnia magna* showed a no-observed-effect concentration (NOEC) of 32 mg/litre for TCPP based on adult mortality. No reproductive effects were seen at lower concentrations (SafePharm, undated/b).

A 48-h LC_{50} of 4.6 mg/litre for *Daphnia magna* was reported using TDCPP (Amgard TDCP), together with a NOEC of 1.8 mg/litre (SafePharm, 1993a).

9.2.3 *Fish*

The 96-h LC_{50} for the fathead minnow (*Pimephales promelas*) was 51 mg/litre (based on measured concentrations; equivalent to 98 mg/litre nominal concentration) under static conditions. The corresponding LC_{50} for bluegill sunfish (*Lepomis macrochirus*) was 180 mg/litre. The NOEC for both species was estimated to be 9.8 mg/litre for TCPP as Antiblaze 80 (Mobil 1985b,c).

The 96-h LC_{50} for rainbow trout (*Oncorhynchus mykiss*) was 1.1 mg/litre for TDCPP (Amgard TDCP) and the NOEC 0.56 mg/litre (SafePharm, 1993b). One out of 6 goldfish (*Carassius auratus*) died after exposure to TDCPP at 1 mg/litre for 168 h and all fish died after exposure to 5 mg/litre (Eldefrawi et al., 1977). The 96-h LC_{50} values for killifish (*Oryzias latipes*) and goldfish (*Carassius auratus*) were reported to be 3.6 and 5.1 mg/litre, respectively, for a static exposure system. Killifish exposed to 3.5 mg/litre for 24 h showed spinal deformities (Sasaki et al., 1981).

9.3 Terrestrial organisms

An acute toxicity test in artificial soil on TDCPP (Amgard TDCP) conducted according to OECD Guideline 207 on the earthworm *Eisenia foetida* gave an LC_{50} value after 14 h of 130 mg/kg soil and a NOEC of 100 mg/kg soil (SafePharm, 1996c). The corresponding values for TCPP (Amgard TMCP) were a 14-h LC_{50} of 97 mg/kg and a NOEC of 32 mg/kg soil (SafePharm, 1996d).

10. EVALUATION

10.1 TCPP

Residues of TCPP are found infrequently and at low concentration in food items. TCPP has not been found in drinking-water. The low volatility of TCPP precludes significant exposure from air. Exposure to TCPP from these sources will not present an acute hazard to the general population. Although toxicological data from long-term studies are limited, because of low exposure to TCPP the risk of adverse health effects to the general population is negligible.

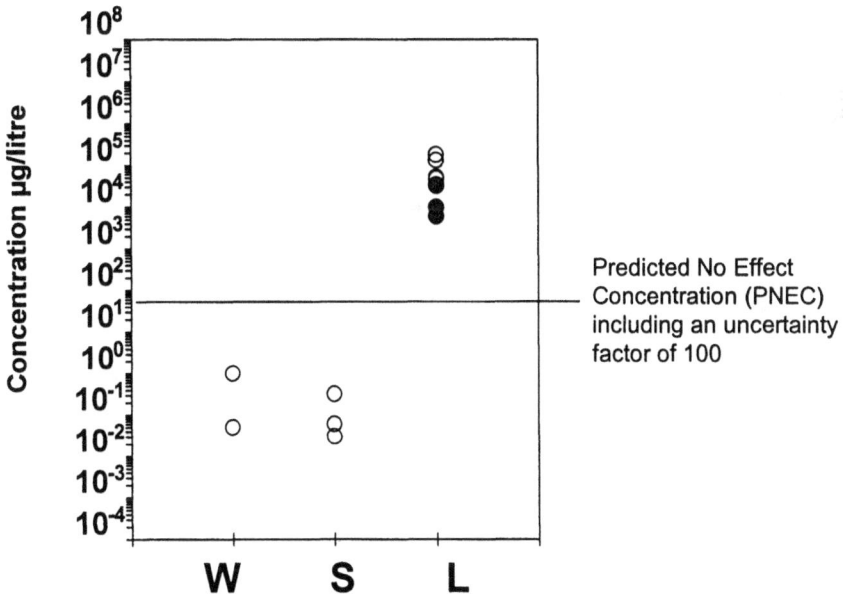

Fig. 1. Plot of measured concentrations in surface waters (W), sewage effluents (s) and reported toxicity values (L) for TCPP (solid symbols are NOECs)

TCPP has been tested at three trophic levels for acute exposure and two trophic levels for chronic exposure of organisms relevant to the environment. The lowest reported chronic NOEC is more than 3 orders of magnitude higher than the highest reported concentration in sewage effluent (Fig. 1). There will be no adverse effects on the environment from the use of TCPP.

10.2 TDCPP

TDCPP has been tested at three trophic levels for acute exposure and two trophic levels for chronic exposure of organisms relevant to the environment. The lowest reported chronic NOEC is more than 3 orders of magnitude higher than the highest reported concentration in sewage effluent and surface waters (Fig. 2). There will be no adverse effects on the environment from the use of TDCPP.

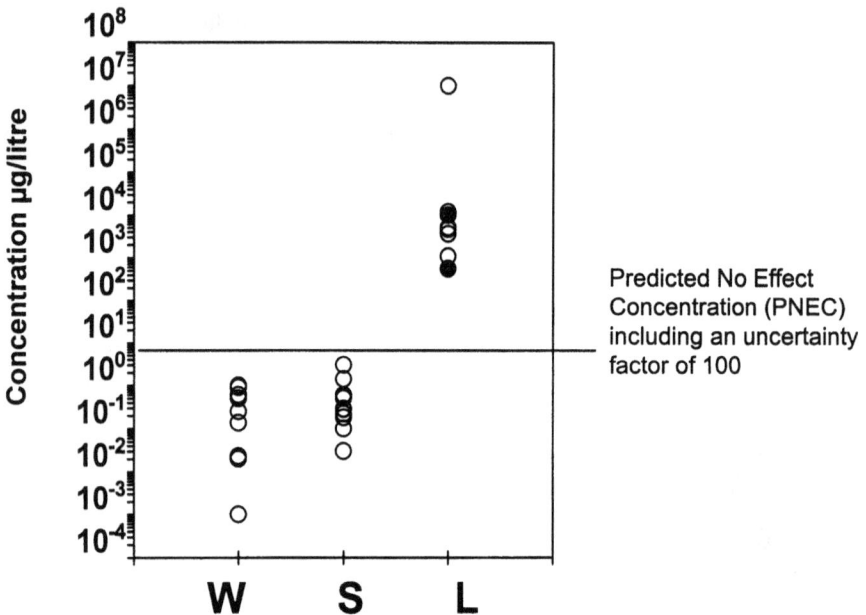

Fig. 2. Plot of measured concentrations in surface waters (W), sewage effluents (S) and reported toxicity values (L) for TDCPP
(solid symbols are NOECs)

Residues of TDCPP are found infrequently and at low concentration in food items and drinking-water. The low volatility of TDCPP precludes significant exposure from air. Exposure to TDCPP from these sources will not present an acute hazard to the general population. TDCPP was genotoxic in bacterial tests and in some *in vitro* mammalian cell tests. However, it has not been sufficiently tested for mutagenicity *in vivo*. TDCPP has been found to be carcinogenic in rats. The mechanism of carcinogenicity has not be elucidated. The exposure level leading to the residues found in humans is unknown. Insufficient information, therefore, is available to estimate accurately human risk. However, because of the low exposure, the risk is expected to be low.

11. FURTHER RESEARCH

Further investigations of the tumorigenicity of TDCPP and the mechanisms underlying it are needed.

TRIS(2-CHLOROETHYL) PHOSPHATE

A1. SUMMARY

Tris(2-chloroethyl) phosphate (TCEP) is a colourless to pale yellow liquid, which is used as a flame retardant mainly in the production of liquid unsaturated polyester resins. It is also used in textile back-coating formulations, PVC compounds, cellulose ester compounds and coatings. It is not volatile and its solubility in water is 8 g/litre. It is soluble in most organic solvents. Its log octanol/water partition coefficient is 1.7.

Analysis is by GC/MS. Concentration of TCEP from water prior to analysis can be achieved using XAD resin or activated charcoal, followed by extraction with various organic solvents.

TCEP is manufactured from phosphorus oxychloride and ethylene oxide. Production and use of TCEP has been in decline since the 1980s. Annual worldwide demand was less than 4000 tonnes in 1997.

TCEP is not readily biodegradable. Bioconcentration factors are low and the half-life of elimination in fish is 0.7 h.

Traces of TCEP have been detected in river water, seawater, drinking-water, sediment, biota (fish and shellfish) and in a few samples of various foods.

In rats, oral doses of TCEP are absorbed and distributed around the body to various organs, particularly the liver and kidney, but also the brain. Metabolites in rats and mice include bis(2-chloroethyl) carboxymethyl phosphate; bis(2-chloroethyl) hydrogen phosphate; and bis(2-chloroethyl)-2-hydroxyethyl phosphate glucuronide. Excretion is rapid, nearly complete and mainly via the urine.

TCEP is of low to moderate acute oral toxicity (oral LD_{50} in the rat = 1150 mg/kg body weight).

In repeat dose studies, TCEP caused adverse effects on the brain (hippocampal lesions in rats), liver and kidneys. The NOEL was 22 mg/kg body weight per day and the LOEL 44 mg/kg body weight per day for increased weights of liver and kidneys in rats.

TCEP is non-irritant to skin and eyes, but has not been tested for sensitization potential.

TCEP is not teratogenic. It adversely affects the fertility of male rats and mice.

No conclusions can be drawn about the mutagenicity of TCEP as *in vitro* test results were inconsistent and an *in vivo* bone marrow micronucleus test gave equivocal results.

TCEP causes benign and malignant tumours at various organ sites in rats and mice.

A very high oral dose of TCEP caused some inhibition of plasma cholinesterase and brain neuropathy target esterase in hens, but did not cause delayed neurotoxicity. In rats, a high dose of TCEP caused convulsions, brain lesions and impaired performance in a water maze.

The LC_{50}/EC_{50} values for organisms in the environment range from 90 to 5000 mg/litre.

A2. IDENTITY, PHYSICAL AND CHEMICAL PROPERTIES, AND ANALYTICAL METHODS

A2.1 Identity

Chemical formula: $C_6H_{12}Cl_3O_4P$

Chemical structure:

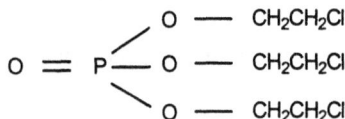

Relative molecular mass: 285.49

CAS name: tris(2-chloroethyl) phosphate

CAS registry number: 115-96-8

IUPAC name: phosphoric acid, tris(2-chloroethyl) ester

Synonyms: phosphoric acid, tris(2-chloroethyl) ester;
                        tris(beta chloroethyl) phosphate;
                        tris(chloroethyl) phosphate;
                        tris(2-chloroethyl) phosphate;
                        tris(2-chloroethyl) orthophosphate;
                        2-chloroethanol phosphate (3:1);
                        ethanol, 2-chlorophosphate (3:1)

Trade names: Celanese Celluflex CEF; Celluflex CEF;
                        Disflamoll TCA; Fyrol CEF; Fyrol CF;
                        Genomoll P; Niax 3CF; Niax Flame
                        retardant 3 (nospaa)CF; Hosta flam
                        UP 810; Amgard TCEP; Tolgard TCEP;
                        Antiblaze TCEP; Levagard EP; Nuogard
                        TCEP

Common name: TCEP

A2.2 Physical and chemical properties

TCEP is a clear, colourless to pale yellow liquid with a slight odour.

Boiling point:	351 °C (at 760 mmHg)
Specific gravity:	1.425 at 20 °C
Solubility:	slightly soluble in water (8 g/litre at 20 °C); soluble in aliphatic hydrocarbons, polar organic solvents such as alcohols, esters, ketones, and in aromatic hydrocarbons and chlorinated hydrocarbons
Vapour pressure:	< 10 mmHg at 25 °C
Flash point:	202 °C (Pensky Martin closed cup)
Stability:	Rapid decomposition occurs above 220 °C; stable to short-term exposure at 150 °C. The products of thermal decomposition are carbon monoxide, hydrogen chloride, 2-chloroethane and dichloroethane. Hydrolytic stability decreases with increasing temperature and pressure or extreme pH.
Refractive index:	1.4721 at 20 °C
Viscosity:	34 cP at 25 °C
Henry's law constant:	3.29×10^{-6}
n-Octanol/water partition coefficient (log P_{ow}):	1.7

A2.3 Conversion factors

$1 \text{ mg/m}^3 = 11.68 \text{ ppm}$
$1 \text{ ppm} = 0.0856 \text{ mg/m}^3$

A2.4 Analytical methods

Selected methods for the analysis of TCEP are presented in Table 7.

Table 7. Methods for the analysis of tris(2-chloroethyl) phosphate

Sample matrix	Sample preparation	Assay procedure[a]	Limit of detection	References
Air	Sample on glass-fibre filter or XAD-7 resin; prefractionate on silica gel column	GC/NPD	0.04–0.1 ng	Haraguchi et al. (1985)
Water	Extract with dichloromethane; dry (anhydrous sodium sulfate); concentrate	GC/MS	10 ng/litre	Ishikawa et al. (1985a); Ishikawa & Baba (1988)
	Extract with dichloromethane	GC/FPD	2 ng/litre	Burchill et al. (1983)
Drinking-water	Adsorb on XAD resin cartridge; extract with dichloromethane; dry (anhydrous sodium sulfate); concentrate	GC/NPD	0.3 ng/litre[b]	LeBel et al. (1981)
	Adsorb on XAD resin cartridge; elute with acetone/ hexane; dry (anhydrous sodium sulfate); concentrate; extract (dichloromethane)	GC/MS and GC/NPD	0.1 ng/litre	LeBel et al. (1987)
Sediment	Extract with acetone; filter; add filtrate to purified water, extract with dichloromethane; dry (anhydrous sodium sulfate); concentrate	GC/MS	5 ng/g	Ishikawa et al. (1985a)
Seawater, fish, sea sediment	Extract with acetonitrile and dichloromethane; adsorb; extract on activated charcoal column; extract with sulfuric acid; wash with sodium hydroxide; purify by Florisil chromatography	GC/MS GC/FPD	1–5 ng/g (fish)	Kenmotsu et al. (1980b)

[a] GC/NPD = gas chromatography/nitrogen phosphorus detection; GC/MS = gas chromatography/ mass spectrometry; GC/FPD = gas chromatography/flame photometric detection.
[b] By direct fortification, in the concentration range of 1 up to 100 ng/litre, a recovery of 90% was obtained.

A3. SOURCES OF HUMAN AND ENVIRONMENTAL EXPOSURE

A3.1 Natural occurrence

TCEP is not a natural product.

A3.2 Anthropogenic sources

A3.2.1 Production and processes

TCEP production and use has been in rapid decline since the 1980s as its historic use in rigid and flexible polyurethane foams and systems has been substituted by other flame retardants.

Global TCEP consumption peaked at over 9000 tonnes in 1989 but had declined to below 4000 tonnes by 1997.

All commercial TCEP has been produced by the reaction of phosphorus oxychloride with ethylene oxide followed by subsequent purification (personal communication by EFRA to IPCS, 1998).

A3.2.2 Uses

Historically TCEP was used in polyurethane foams and systems, mainly for rigid foam but with minor use in flexible polyurethane.

TCEP is currently mainly used in the production of liquid unsaturated polyester resins. It is also used in textile back-coating formulations, PVC compounds, cellulose ester compounds and coatings.

TCEP is not recommended by producers for use as a flame retardant additive for use in textiles nor for use in block polyurethane foams because of the probability of its decomposition (personal communication by EFRA to IPCS, 1998).

A4. ENVIRONMENTAL TRANSPORT, DISTRIBUTION AND TRANSFORMATION

A4.1 Transport and distribution between media

The Henry's law constant has been estimated to be 3.29×10^{-6}, indicating very slow volatilization from surface waters. Estimates for K_{oc} range from 34 to 141, indicating low adsorption to soil or aquatic sediment and, therefore, high mobility of TCEP. It can be assumed that TCEP released to the environment would, therefore, be predominantly in the water compartment (National Medical Library, 1998).

A4.2 Transformation

A4.2.1 Abiotic

TCEP hydrolyses slowly in water. Hydrolysis increases with temperature and at the extremes of the pH range (personal communication by Courtaulds to IPCS).

A4.2.2 Biotic

TCEP has been evaluated as "inherently biodegradable" in tests conducted aerobically under OECD guidelines (ECB, 1995).

There was virtually no uptake of TCEP into killifish (*Oryzias latipes*) or goldfish (*Carassius auratus*) over a 100-h period and, consequently, little metabolism of the compound (Sasaki et al., 1981).

A4.3 Bioaccumulation

Bioconcentration factors (BCF) of 1.4–2.2 were measured for killifish (*Oryzias latipes*) exposed to TCEP concentrations of 0.3–8.5 mg/litre for 96 h. BCF values for the same species, exposed for 5 or 11 days to concentrations of 12.7 or 2.3 mg/litre, respectively, in continuous-flow systems, were 1.1 and 1.3, respectively. The half-life for elimination in clean water following continuous-flow exposure was 0.7 h (Sasaki et al., 1982).

Goldfish (*Carassius auratus*) exposed to TCEP at 4 mg/litre for 96 h under static conditions showed a BCF of 0.9 (Sasaki et al., 1981).

A5. ENVIRONMENTAL LEVELS AND HUMAN EXPOSURE

A5.1 Environmental levels

A5.1.1 Air

No data on the levels of TCEP in air are available.

A5.1.2 Water

A5.1.2.1 Surface water

Water samples were analysed in 1975 and 1978 in Japan for TCEP. In 1975, 8/40 water samples contained 0.1–0.34 µg TCEP/litre (limit of determination, 0.013–0.1 µg/litre). In 1978 the values were 0.09 µg/litre (limit of determination, 0.01–1 µg/litre) for 3/114 water samples (Environmental Agency Japan, 1983, 1987).

A 1980 survey around Kitakyushu, Japan, identified TCEP in 14/16 samples at levels in the range of 0.017–0.347 µg/litre in river water and in 9/9 samples (0.014–0.060 µg/litre) of seawater (limit of detection 10 ng/litre) (Ishikawa et al., 1985a). TCEP was also detected in river water and sewage sludge from the Okayama area (Kenmochi et al., 1981).

In Canadian rivers at 13 sites, TCEP was found at a mean concentration of 0.0087 µg/litre. Water from the Great Lakes contained TCEP at a mean concentration of 0.0017 µg/litre at 10 Canadian sites (US EPA, 1988).

TCEP was detected in water from the River Rhine at Lobith in the Netherlands at 1 µg/litre in 1979 (Zoeteman, 1980) and at levels from 0.16 to 0.35 µg/litre in 1986 (Brauch & Kühn, 1988). The compound was also found in the Dutch river Waal in 1974 (Meijers & van der Leer, 1976). In Italy, Galassi (1991) reported concentration ranging from < 10 up to 293 ng/litre at one river station (River Po) and two marine stations in the Adriatic Sea in sample collected at three periods in 1988. Barcelo et al. (1990) identified TCEP in a Spanish river

(Llobregat) in May and June 1988 at concentrations of 0.4 and 0.3 µg/litre, respectively.

TCEP was detected at levels of up to 5.5 µg/litre in raw water samples from the River Trent, United Kingdom, in 1979–1980 (Burchill et al., 1983).

A5.1.2.2 Drinking-water

In a study of drinking-water from surface supplies in Northern Italy, Galassi et al. (1989) found TCEP at concentrations between 0.01 µg/litre and 0.04 µg/litre.

TCEP has also been identified in drinking-water from Canada; 0.0003–0.0092 µg/litre in six eastern Ontario treatment plants in 1978 (LeBel et al., 1981); 0.0002–0.052 µg/litre in 22 of 29 municipalities in 1979 (Williams & LeBel, 1981); 0.0003–0.0138 µg/litre in 11 of 12 Great Lakes municipalities in 1980 (Williams et al., 1982); and 0.003–0.0096 µg/litre in 1982 and 1983 in four out of five Great Lakes areas (LeBel et al., 1987).

Drinking-water was collected at six Great Lakes water treatment plants from Eastern Ontario, Canada and analysed for TCEP. From each plant two samples were taken. The concentrations ranged from 0.6 to 3.7 ng/litre as determined by GC/MS; determination by GC/NPD showed concentrations of 3.0 up to 9.6 ng/litre (LeBel et al., 1987).

In the USA, 15 pooled drinking-water samples contained an average of 0.0026 µg/litre (US EPA, 1988).

Drinking-water was collected in Japan over a period of 1 year and a mean concentration of 0.0174 (range 0.002–0.060) µg/litre was found (Adachi et al., 1984) (no details).

In a survey of infant and toddler dietary intake conducted in the USA from October 1978 to September 1979, 1 sample of drinking-water containing 0.3 µg TCEP/litre was identified (Gartrell et al., 1985a).

A5.1.2.3 Effluents

Industrial and domestic wastewater effluents in Kitakyushu, Japan, contained detectable levels of TCEP (limit of determination, 0.03 µg/litre). Concentrations were not detectable (ND) to 0.087 µg/litre at 3 food factories, 0.043–0.74 µg/litre at 8 chemical factories, ND to 14.0 µg/litre at 5 steel factories, ND to 11.0 µg/litre at 6 other industrial sites, and 0.5–1.2 µg/litre in effluent (0.54 to 1.2 in influent) at 5 sewage treatment plants. Concentrations in river water samples ranged from ND to 0.35 µg/litre (limit of determination 0.01 µg/litre) (Ishikawa et al., 1985b).

A5.1.2.4 Leachates

Oman & Hynning (1993) using GC-MS (detection limit 1–10 µg/litre) showed the presence of TCEP in one sample of a municipal landfill leachate.

TCEP was identified at a mean concentration of 0.57 µg/litre in two monitoring wells adjacent to a municipal wastewater infiltration system at Fort Devens (near Boston), Massachusetts, USA (Bedient et al., 1983).

A5.2 Sediment

Sediment samples were analysed for TCEP in 1975 and 1978 in Japan. In 1975, 1/20 sediment samples contained 0.07 mg/kg (limit of determination, 0.025 mg/kg). In 1978, 114 sediment samples did not contain TCEP (limit of determination, 0.001–0.05 mg/kg) (Environmental Agency Japan, 1983, 1987).

A survey conducted in Japan in 1977 and 1978 did not detect TCEP in 99 samples of sediment from rivers, estuaries or the sea. In 1980, however, 5/6 samples taken around Kitakyushu showed TCEP at concentrations of 0.013–0.028 µg/kg sediment (limit of detection 5 ng/kg) (Ishikawa et al., 1985a).

A5.3 Biota and food

A5.3.1 Biota

Fish samples collected in Japan in 1975 and 1978 were analysed. In 1975 20 fish samples did not contain TCEP (limit of determination 0.025 mg/kg), but in 1978 9/93 fish samples contained 0.005–0.14 mg/kg (limit of determination 0.001–0.05 mg/kg) (Environmental Agency Japan, 1983, 1987).

TCEP was found at levels ranging between < 0.005 and 0.019 mg/kg in fish and shellfish sampled in the Okayama area (Kenmochi et al., 1981).

A5.3.2 Food

When fruit and fruit juices were sampled for TCEP from ten cities in the USA in 1979, one contained 0.002 mg/kg (Gartrell et al., 1985a,b). In oil and fat from toddler foods sampled from 1980 to 1982 in 13 different US cities, TCEP was found in one sample at a concentration of 0.0385 mg/kg. Over the same period, samples of meat, fish and poultry for adult consumption were collected in 27 different US cities. TCEP was found in one sample at a concentration of 0.0067 mg/kg (Gartrell et al., 1986).

The daily intake of TCEP by infants and toddlers in 1978, 1979, 1980 and 1981/1982 was ND, 0.016, 0.004 and ND µg/kg body weight for infants and ND, 0.009, ND and 0.028 µg/kg body weight for toddlers (Gartrell et al., 1986).

In another survey of infant and toddler diets over the period October 1979 to September 1980, TCEP was found in 1 sample of composite fruit and fruit juice at a concentration of 0.2 µg/litre. It was not detected in other foods tested (Gartrell et al., 1985b).

A6. KINETICS AND METABOLISM IN LABORATORY ANIMALS

A6.1 Mice

In a study on male B6C3F$_1$ mice, more than 70% of an oral dose of 175 mg ^{14}C-labelled TCEP/kg body weight was excreted in urine within 8 h. Identified urinary metabolites of TCEP in mice were bis(2-chloroethyl) carboxymethyl phosphate, bis(2-chloroethyl) hydrogen phosphate and bis(2-chloroethyl) 2-hydroxyethyl phosphate glucuronide (Burka et al., 1991).

A6.2 Rats

Male and female Fischer-344 rats were gavaged with ^{14}C-labelled TCEP at 0, 175, 350 or 700 mg/kg body weight. Plasma concentrations of TCEP and its metabolites in rats dosed at 175 mg/kg peaked by 30 min. Concentrations were higher in females at the peak but by 4 h there were no sex differences. TCEP concentrations in the hippocampus, the site of the major lesions, were no higher than in other brain tissues and there were no sex differences (Herr et al., 1991).

Minegishi et al. (1988) studied the distribution and excretion of ^{14}C-labelled TCEP in 5-week-old male Wistar rats orally dosed with 50 µmol/kg body weight. The label was concentrated by various tissues, especially the liver and kidney, during the first 6 h following administration and then rapidly decreased. Most of the label was excreted by 24 h and by 168 h less than 1% remained in tissues. Urine accounted for 96%, faeces for 6%, and expired air for 2% of the label. Rapid urinary excretion was confirmed by Burka et al. (1991), who found 40% of the label in urine within 8 h after a dose of 175 mg ^{14}C TCEP/kg body weight in male and female rats. They identified the same urinary metabolites as those listed above for mice.

Chapman et al. (1991) found that the hepatic microsomal fraction from male rats, but not female rats, metabolized TCEP. Liver slices and blood plasma, however, of both sexes metabolized the compound, demonstrating that at least part of the metabolism is extramicrosomal.

Liver slices and microsomes from both male and female humans metabolized TCEP, but plasma and whole blood did not.

Urinary elimination of TCEP in rats was not increased by 9 daily doses of 175 mg/kg, indicating that TCEP is not capable of inducing its own metabolism (Burka et al., 1991).

A7. EFFECTS ON LABORATORY MAMMALS AND *IN VITRO* TEST SYSTEMS

A7.1 Single exposure

The acute oral LD_{50} for TCEP was 1.23 g/kg body weight following a 30-day observation period in rats. An oral LD_{50} of 0.5 g/kg body weight was found in a second study with male rats. Treated rats died within 24 h and showed spasmodic contractions and acute depressions. The LD_{50} values for female rats were reported to be 0.79, 0.50 and 0.43 g/kg body weight with three different lots of the chemical (Ulsamer et al., 1980). Smyth et al. (1951) reported an LD_{50} of 1.41 g/kg body weight in rats.

In a study conducted according to OECD Test Guidelines 401, groups of 5 male and 5 female Sprague-Dawley rats received 800, 1000 or 1260 mg/kg body weight by oral gavage. One female receiving 1000 mg/kg died on day 2 and 4/5 males and 4/5 females receiving 1260 mg/kg body weight died by day 4. The LD_{50} was calculated to be 1150 mg/kg body weight. Clinical signs of toxicity included piloerection and increased salivation amongst all animals; hunched posture, abnormal gait, lethargy, laboured respiration, ptosis and pale extremities were observed amongst all animals receiving 1000 and 1260 mg/kg body weight. No clinical signs of toxicity were observed in surviving animals from day 4 onwards. No microscopic pathology abnormalities were seen amongst decedent animals or those killed on completion of the 14-day observation period (Kynoch & Denton, 1990)

In an earlier study conducted at the same location, male and female CD rats (5 animals per group) received 2.5, 3.2, 4.0 and 5.0 g/kg body weight by oral gavage. Signs of reaction to treatment observed in all animals within one half-hour of dosing were pilo-erection, hunched posture, abnormal gait and increased salivation. The calculated LD_{50} was 3.6 g/kg body weight for males and females combined (Gardner, 1987).

A7.2 Short-term exposure

A7.2.1 Mice

Groups of five B6C3F$_1$ mice of each sex were gavaged with 0, 44, 88, 175, 350 or 700 mg TCEP/kg body weight in corn oil 5 days/week for 2 weeks. Mice given 350 and 700 mg/kg exhibited ataxia and convulsive movements during the first 3 days of dosing. No changes of body weight gain, absolute and relative organ weight or histopathological abnormalities were observed (US NTP, 1990; Matthews et al., 1990).

A7.2.2 Rats

A 30-day feeding study, in which up to 0.5% of TCEP was given in the diet to male and female rats, resulted in no adverse effects on growth, appearance and behaviour, liver and kidney weights or changes in pathological examinations of survivors (Ulsamer et al., 1980).

Groups of five rats of each sex of the strain F-344/N were administered by gavage 0, 22, 44, 88, 175 or 350 mg TCEP/kg body weight 5 days/week for 2 weeks. No difference in body weight gain was found in the treated animals versus controls. The mean absolute and relative kidney weights of the males given 175 and 350 mg/kg body weight were increased (10% and 12%, respectively). Liver weights of the high-dose females were also significantly increased (17%). Serum cholinesterase activity was not reduced in males, but was decreased by 18% and 20% in female at 175 and 350 mg/kg body weight. No gross or histopathological abnormalities were found (US NTP, 1990; Matthews et al., 1990).

A7.3 Long-term exposure

A7.3.1 Mice

Groups of 10 male and 10 female B6C3F$_1$ mice (9–10 weeks old) were administered by gavage 0, 44, 88, 175, 350 or 700 TCEP mg/kg body weight in corn oil 5 days/week for 16 weeks. During week 4, the two highest doses were incorrectly prepared and administered for the first 3 days of this week. The mice of the two highest dose levels received double the target levels. No difference in body weight gain or serum cholinesterase activity was found between the treated groups and the control group. The absolute liver weights were significantly increased (P ≤ 0.01) in females receiving 175, 375 and 700 mg/kg body weight (14%, 20% and 13%, respectively) and in males receiving 700 mg/kg (5%). The liver-to-body weight ratios, however, were not increased. Male mice in the 175, 350 and 700 mg/kg body weight groups had significantly (P ≤ 0.01) reduced absolute kidney weights (5%, 10% and 20%, respectively). The kidney-to-body weight ratio, however, was not affected. No gross abnormalities were observed, but epithelial cells with enlarged nuclei (mild cytomegaly and karyo-megaly) were observed in the renal tubules in all animals given 700 mg/kg body weight. The lesions were observed primarily in the proximal convoluted tubules of the inner cortex and outer strip of the outer medulla and to a lesser extent in the straight portion of the loops of Henle in the medulla (US NTP, 1990; Matthews et al., 1990).

A7.3.2 Rats

Groups of 10 male and 10 female F-344/N rats (8–9 weeks old) were administered 0, 22, 44, 88, 175 or 350 TCEP mg/kg body weight in corn oil by gavage, 5 days/week for 16 weeks (females) and 18 weeks (males). The animals with the two highest dose levels received a double dose for 3 days in week 4. Consequently two females of each dose level died and a few other animals showed signs of intoxication; ataxia, excessive salivation, gasping and convulsions. During the 16-week exposure additional animals died in these two groups; the deaths of one male of the 175 mg/kg body weight group and 4 males and 3 females of the 350 mg/kg body weight group were attributed to chemical toxicity. Body weight was comparable with the controls. The relative liver and kidney weights were significantly (P ≤ 0.01) increased in the high-dose males and in females receiving 44 to 350 mg/kg body weight. In males given 350 mg/kg per day the increases in relative liver and kidney weights were 22% and 26%, respectively. In females the increases in relative liver weight were 13%, 13%, 19% and 50% in the 44, 88, 175 and 350 mg/kg body weight groups, respectively; the increases in relative kidney weight were 8%, 11%, 11% and 22% in the 44, 88, 175 and 350 mg/kg groups, respectively.

Cholinesterase activity determined in serum at necropsy was 75% and 59% of the control value at 175 and 350 mg/kg body weight, respectively, in female rats, but was not reduced in males. No gross lesions were observed, but necrosis of neurons, mainly of the dorsomedial portion of the pyramidal row of the hippocampus, was observed in 10/10 females and 2/10 males of the 350 mg/kg group and in 8/10 females of the 175 mg/kg group. Mineral deposits were present in the affected areas of the brain. In the high-dose females, neuronal necrosis was seen in the thalamus. Based on the increases in relative liver and kidney weights in females, the NOEL in this study was 22 mg/kg per day and the LOEL 44 mg/kg per day (US NTP, 1990; Matthews et al., 1990)

A7.4 Skin and eye irritation or sensitization

A7.4.1 Skin irritation

In a study conducted according to modern protocol standards, 0.5 ml TCEP was applied to the skin of three New Zealand white rabbits under a semi-occlusive dressing for 4 h. Slight erythema (grade 1) was observed in each animal on day 1 only. Thereafter there were no signs of skin irritation (Liggett & McRae, 1991c).

A7.4.2 Eye irritation

In a study conducted according to modern protocol standards, 0.1 ml TCEP was instilled into the eye of each of 3 New Zealand white rabbits (Liggett & McRae, 1991d). Slight conjunctival redness (grade 1) was observed in each animal on day 1 and in one animal on day 2. Thereafter, there were no signs of eye irritation.

A7.4.3 Sensitization

No data on the possible sensitizing effects of TCEP are available.

A7.5 Reproductive toxicity, embryotoxicity and teratogenicity

A7.5.1 Developmental toxicity

Development toxicity was tested by the Chernoff/Kavlock preliminary development toxicity test by treating pregnant CD-1 mice on gestation days 6–15 at an overtly maternally toxic dose of TCEP.

The dose used was 940 mg/kg per day. The depression in maternal body weight gain was 12%. There were no significant adverse effects on maternal mortality, pup survival rate, litter size, weight gain of pups, or birth weight of pups (Hardin, 1987; Hardin et al., 1987).

Wistar rats were given by gavage 50, 100 or 200 mg TCEP/kg body weight suspended in olive oil on days 7–15 of gestation. No change in maternal body weight gain, food consumption or general appearance was found in the low- and mid-dose groups. In the high-dose group, maternal food consumption was markedly suppressed; piloerection and general weakness occurred and 7/30 dams died. On day 20 of gestation, no increase in fetal death or malformations attributable to treatment were observed in any group. There was some increase (not statistically significant) in the incidence of super-numerary cervical and lumbar ribs in the high-dose group (this end-point is considered a variation not a malformation). Postnatal examination revealed normal development in the offspring of all groups; no abnormalities on morphological examination or in functional behaviour tests (open field, water maze, rota rod, inclined plane test, pain reflex or Preyer's reflex) were found (Kawashima et al., 1983a,b).

A7.5.2 *Fertility*

In a study in B6C3F$_1$ mice, animals were dosed by gavage at dose levels of 44, 175 and 700 mg/kg body weight for 13 weeks. In the males, no effects were noted regarding body weight, absolute and relative cauda weights, relative epididymis weight, motility or sperm concentration. The absolute epididymis weight and absolute and relative testes weights were decreased and an increase in the number of sperm with abnormal morphology were noted. In the females, no increase in estrous cycle length was noted in any of the treatment groups (Morrissey et al., 1988).

TCEP was tested for its effects on fertility and reproduction in Swiss CD-1 mice according to a continuous breeding protocol. Animals were exposed via gavage to doses of 175, 350 and 700 mg/kg body weight. Males and females (F$_0$ generation) were exposed daily for 7 days pre-cohabitation and 98 days cohabitation periods. In the F$_0$ generation, TCEP decreased the number of litters per pair and the number of live pups per litter. Both sexes were affected, but the males were relatively more sensitive. All sperm end-points (concentration, motility and percentage of abnormal sperm) were adversely affected. Due to poor fertility in the 700 mg/kg body weight per day group, only one F_0 pair delivered a litter. None of these pups survived to postnatal day 4. The data indicated reduced fertility due to TCEP exposure at doses of 175 mg/kg body weight or more (Gulati et al., 1991).

In a study on F-344 rats, animals were dosed by gavage at levels of 22, 88 and 175 mg/kg body weight for 13 weeks. In the males no effects were noted on body weight, absolute and relative cauda weights, absolute and relative epididymal weights, absolute and relative testes weights, sperm concentration, and number of abnormal sperm. However, sperm motility was reduced. In the females, no increase in estrous cycle length was noted in any of the treatment groups (Morrissey et al., 1988).

In an inhalation study using whole body exposure, male rats (strain and group size not specified) were continuously exposed to 0.5 or 1.5 mg TCEP/m^3 for 4 months. Testicular toxicity was seen at both dose levels, with most severe effects at the highest dose. There were decreased sperm counts, decreased sperm mortality and abnormal sperm morphology. Histology of the testes showed an increased number of spermatogonia but decreased numbers of sperm in the later stages of development. When the treated males were mated, there was decreased fertility at the 1.5 mg/m^3 dose, with increased pre- and post-implantation loss, and litter sizes were decreased (Shepel'skaya & Dyshinevich, 1981).

A7.6 Mutagenicity and related end-points

A7.6.1 In vitro *studies*

TCEP was found not to be mutagenic in *Salmonella typhimurium* strains TA1535, TA1537, TA1538, TA98 and TA100 at dose levels up to 5 mg/plate, both with and without metabolic activation with Aroclor 1254-induced rat liver S9 (Simmon et al., 1977).

Negative results were obtained when TCEP was tested at doses of 3.3, 10, 33, 100 and 333 µg/plate in liquid pre-incubation assays employing *Salmonella typhimurium* TA1535, TA1537, TA98 and

TA100, both with and without a metabolic system from Aroclor 1254-induced rat liver or Syrian hamster liver S9 (Haworth et al., 1983).

In contrast, TCEP at dose levels of 285, 755, 2850 and 8550 µg/plate produced a dose-related increase in mutations (with a maximum 7.6-fold increase of revertants over the control at 2850 µg/plate) in *Salmonella typhimurium* TA1535 in the presence but not in the absence of metabolic system from Kanechlor 500-induced Wistar rat liver S9. The same doses produced a dose-related increase in mutations in TA100 with a maximum 1.8-fold increase in revertants at 2850 µg/plate (Nakamura et al., 1979).

TCEP (5 to 1600 µg/ml) was tested for CA and SCE in Chinese hamster ovary cells both with and without an exogenous metabolism system from liver of Sprague-Dawley rats induced by Aroclor 1254. TCEP did not induce CAs. The results of the SCE test were regarded as equivocal because a positive response was seen only in one trial with S9 fraction at 500 and 1600 µg/ml but was not observed in a repeated trial under the same conditions (Galloway et al., 1987).

The frequency of 6-thioguanine-resistant mutants using V79 cells without S9 was determined at 0, 500, 1000 and 2000 µg/ml. TCEP did not significantly increase the number of 6-thioguanine-resistant mutants (Sala et al., 1982).

TCEP was tested for SCEs in V79 cells in two separate experiments at concentration levels of 343, 490, 700 and 1000 µg/ml (exp. I) and 2000 and 3000 (exp. II). In the first experiment, a statistical increase in the number of SCEs was noted at 700 and 1000 µg/ml with S9 (3-methylcholanthrene-induced rat liver) and at 700 µg/ml without S9 (1000 µg/ml was not tested without S9). In the second experiment, TCEP was only tested without S9 and was positive at both concentrations tested. However, the 3000 µg/ml concentration caused cytotoxicity (Sala et al., 1982).

In the presence of S9 from livers of Wistar rats induced with methylcholanthrene, TCEP at 900 and 1500 µg/ml gave a negative result in a transformation assay using C3H10T1/2 cells.

A high level of transformation of Syrian hamster embryo cells was observed with TCEP at concentrations of 400 and 500 µg/ml. The two highest dose concentrations (600 and 800 µg/ml) were toxic and no transformation was seen at these concentrations (Sala et al., 1982).

TCEP caused a dose-related (343–1000 µg/ml) increase in the incidence of sister chromatid exchange in the Chinese hamster V79 cell line, but doses from 500 to 2000 µg/ml did not induce mutations at the HPRT locus in the same cell line (Sala et al., 1982).

A7.6.2 In vivo *studies*

TCEP was administered intraperitoneally at dose levels of 63.5, 125, 250 mg/kg body weight to groups of male and female Chinese hamsters. There was no clear dose-dependent increase in the number of micronuclei isolated from bone marrow cells. However, in some of the dose groups an approximate doubling in the number of micronuclei was noted (females at 62.5 and 125 mg/kg body weight, and males at 250 mg/kg body weight) (Sala et al., 1982).

TCEP gave a negative response in the w/w+ bioassay for somatic cell damage in *Drosophila melanogaster* (Vogel & Nivard, 1993).

A7.7 Carcinogenicity

A7.7.1 Oral

A7.7.1.1 Mice

Groups of 50 male and 50 female Slc:ddy mice received approximately 0, 12, 60, 300 or 1500 mg/kg body weight per day by dietary administration (assuming 30 g body weight and 3 g/day food consumption) for 18 months (Takada et al., 1989). Distension of the abdomen was noted in males receiving 1500 mg/kg per day from week 65. Reduced survival was noted in males and females receiving 1500 mg/kg per day (approximately 40% survival compared to around 65% survival in controls). A marked reduction in body weight gain was noted in males and females receiving 1500 mg/kg per day (approximately 60% lower than the control value). Other groups were not adversely affected, and there were no changes in food consumption. There were no significant changes in haematological parameters recorded at termination. Histologically, hyperplasia, hypertrophy and karyomegaly were observed in the kidney of all treated animals although the incidence and severity of effects in the kidneys was unclear. In addition, cysts of the kidneys, necrosis and interstitial fibrosis were reported only amongst animals given 1500 mg/kg per day, although no further details were available. An increased incidence of renal adenomas was noted in males (0/50, 0/49, 0/49, 2/49, 9/50) and females (0/49, 0/49, 0/50, 0/49, 2/50). In addition, there was an increased incidence of renal carcinomas in males (2/50, 0/49, 2/49, 3/47, 32/50) and females (1/50 at 1500 mg/kg per day and zero in all other groups). In the liver, there was an increased incidence of adenomas in males and females (3/50, 4/49, 3/49, 10/47, 16/50 in males, and 2/50 in females at 1500 mg/kg per day with zero in all other groups). In addition, there was a slight, but not dose-related, increase in the incidence of liver carcinomas in males (1/50, 1/49, 4/49, 2/47, 3/50). A slight increase in the incidence of forestomach papillomas and carcinomas was reported in treated males and females.

Groups of 60 males and 60 females B6C3F$_1$ mice received 0, 175 or 350 mg/kg 5 days/week by gavage for 103 weeks (US NTP, 1990). An interim sacrifice was performed on groups of 10 males and 10 females. At 66 weeks, there were no effects seen on body weight gain, haematology or clinical chemistry. At 103 weeks there were no adverse effects on survival or body weight gain. Non-neoplastic lesions were seen in the kidney; karyomegaly in the proximal convoluted tubules (2/50, 16/50 and 39/50 in males and 0/50, 5/49 and 44/50 in females). In the liver, an increased incidence of eosinophilic foci was observed in males (0/50, 3/50, 8/50). Neoplastic lesions in the kidney were observed: adenoma, 1/50, 0/50 and 1/50 in males and 0/50, 1/49 and 0/50 in females; adenocarcinoma, 0/50, 0/50 and 1/50 in males. In the liver of males an increased incidence of adenomas was seen: 20/50, 18/50 and 28/50. In addition, there was a slight increase in the incidence of Harderian gland adenomas in females.

A7.7.1.2 Rats

Groups of 60 males and 60 females F-344 rats received 0, 44 or 88 mg/kg 5 days/week by gavage for 103 weeks (US NTP, 1990). An interim sacrifice was performed on groups of 10 males and 10 females. At 66 weeks, there were no adverse effects seen on body weight gain or haematology. There were unquantified decreases in serum alkaline phosphatase and alanine aminotransferase in females receiving 88 mg/kg per day. Slight increases in liver and kidney weights were recorded in males at 88 mg/kg per day (14% and 20%, respectively, greater than controls). Also observed at this time point were renal tubule adenomas in one male receiving 88 mg/kg per day and local necrosis and accumulation of inflammatory cells in the cerebrum and thalamus of the brains of 3/10 females given 88 mg/kg per day.

At 103 weeks there were no adverse effects on body weight gain and no clinical signs of toxicity. Reduced survival was noted in males and females at 88 mg/kg per day (males 51% survival compared to 78% in controls; females 37% compared to 66% in controls). No organ weight data were presented for this time point. Non-neoplastic findings in the kidneys were hyperplasia: 0/50, 2/50 and 24/50 in males and 0/50, 3/50, 16/50 in females.

A marked increase in the incidence of degenerative lesions of the brain stem and cerebrum (thalamus, hypothalamus and basal ganglia) (such as gliosis, haemorrhage, necrosis and mineralization) was noted at 88 mg/kg per day (occurring in approximately 40% of females at 88 mg/kg per day compared to 2% of controls).

Neoplastic lesions were observed in the kidney; the frequency of adenomas was 1/50, 5/50 and 24/50 in males and 0/50, 2/50, 5/50 in females. In the brain, benign granular cell tumours were observed in 3/50 males at 88 mg/kg per day only. There were no treatment-related increases in the incidence of tumours in the brain of females. A slight increase in the incidence of thyroid follicular adenomas was noted in males (1/50, 2/48, 3/50), and of carcinomas in males and females (0/50, 0/48, 2/50 in males; 0/50, 2/50, 3/50 in females).

There were increased occurrences of mononuclear cell leukaemia in males (5/50, 14/50, 13/50) and in females (14/50, 16/50, 20/50). These occurrences, however, were within the range of historical controls (2–44%).

A7.7.2 *Dermal*

A7.7.2.1 *Mice*

There was no significant increase in tumours in female Slc/ddy mice whose shaved skin was treated twice weekly for 79 weeks with ethanol solutions containing 5% or 50% of TCEP. However, the amount of the solution applied to skin was not reported (Takada et al., 1991).

An *in vivo* short-term skin test for sebaceous gland suppression and the induction of epidermal hyperplasia was carried out. Groups of 25 Swiss mice (45 days of age) received dorsal applications on days 1, 3 and 5 of TCEP at 0, 31.9, 53.2 and 74.5 mg (total dose applied in three applications). Benzo(*a*)pyrene was used as positive control. TCEP did not suppress the sebaceous gland and did not induce hyperplasia (Sala et al., 1982).

Groups of Swiss mice were used to test TCEP for skin initiation and/or promoter activity. TCEP showed no significant complete carcinogenic, initiating or promoter activity on mouse skin (Sala et al., 1982). A working group of IARC (1990) noted that the promoting activity and complete carcinogenicity of TCEP in the Sala et al. (1982) study could not be evaluated because of the lack of control.

A7.8 Other special studies

A7.8.1 Neurotoxicity

The neurotoxicity effects of TCEP were evaluated in adult (12–14 months old) White Leghorn hens given 14 200 mg/kg body weight of the chemical in corn oil followed 3 weeks later by a second dose. Four out of 18 treated hens died within 6 weeks of the first dose. Egg production ceased, body weights fell and feather loss began shortly after the first treatment. No microscopic changes in brain, spinal cord or sciatic nerve were found after the treatment. In a separate group of hens, the activities of brain neuropathy target esterase and plasma cholinesterase were determined 24 h after the first dose of TCEP. Plasma cholinesterase activity was inhibited by 87% and brain neuropathy target esterase by 30%. No delayed neurotoxicity was observed (Sprague et al., 1981).

White Leghorn hens (12 months old) were orally exposed to 420 mg TECP/kg body weight per day for 5 consecutive days. After 21 days of observation there was no signs of neurotoxicity as compared with TDCP (positive control) which induced an inability to walk, hypertension, ataxia and prostration (Bullock & Kamienski, 1972).

Female Fischer-344 rats gavaged with 275 mg TCEP/kg body weight convulsed within 60–90 min and had extensive loss of CA1 hippocampal pyramidal cells when examined after 7 days. When convulsions were controlled, the histological lesions were diminished, indicating possibly that the lesions were due to convulsions and not directly due to TCEP. In a second study, rats gavaged with 275 mg/kg TCEP body weight had impaired acquisition of a reference memory task in a water maze when trained and tested starting 3 weeks following exposure, suggesting long-term impairment of some brain functions (Tilson et al., 1990).

A8. EFFECTS ON HUMANS

No data concerning the effects of TCEP on humans are available.

A9. EFFECTS ON OTHER ORGANISMS IN THE LABORATORY AND FIELD

A9.1 Microorganisms

The toxicity of TCEP to aerobic bacteria (*Pseudomonas putida*) and anaerobic bacterial cultures from sewage sludge is very low with LC_{50} values in excess of 5000 mg/litre (Bayer, 1986) and 1000 mg/litre (Hoechst, 1985), respectively.

A9.2 Aquatic organisms

A9.2.1 Algae

The EC_{50} for growth of *Tetrahymena pyriformis* was reported to be 126 mg/litre (Yoshioka et al., 1986)

A9.2.2 Invertebrates

Yoshioka et al. (1986) reported an LC_{50} of 1000 mg/litre for a daphnid (*Moina macropoda*) and an LC_{50} of 158 mg/litre for a flatworm (*Dugesia japonica*).

A9.2.3 Fish

Sasaki et al. (1981) reported 96-h LC_{50} values for killifish (*Oryzias latipes*) and goldfish (*Carassius auratus*) of 210 and 90 mg/litre, respectively. Killifish exposed to TCEP at 200 mg/litre for 72 h showed spinal deformities. Yoshioka et al. (1986) reported an LC_{50} for the killifish (*Oryzias latipes*) of 251 mg/litre.

Unpublished studies gave the following acute toxicity values for fish: 48-h LC_{50} for killifish (*Oryzias latipes*) of 300 mg/litre (MITI, 1992); and 96-h LC_{50} for rainbow trout (*Oncorhynchus mykiss*) of 249 mg/litre (NOEC, 50 mg/litre) (Akzo, 1990).

A10. EVALUATION

Traces of TCEP have been found in food items and drinking-water. The low volatility of TCEP precludes significant exposure from air. Exposure to TCEP from these sources will not present an acute hazard to the general population. The genetic toxicity data are ambiguous. TCEP has been found to be carcinogenic in rats and mice. The mechanism of carcinogenicity has not been elucidated. However, because of the low exposure, the risk of adverse health effects from TCEP to the general population is expected to be very low.

TCEP has been tested at three trophic levels for acute and two trophic levels for chronic exposure of organisms relevant to the environment. The lowest reported chronic NOEC is more than 3 orders of magnitude higher than the highest reported concentration in sewage effluent and surface waters (Fig. 3). There will be no adverse effects on the environment from the use of TCEP.

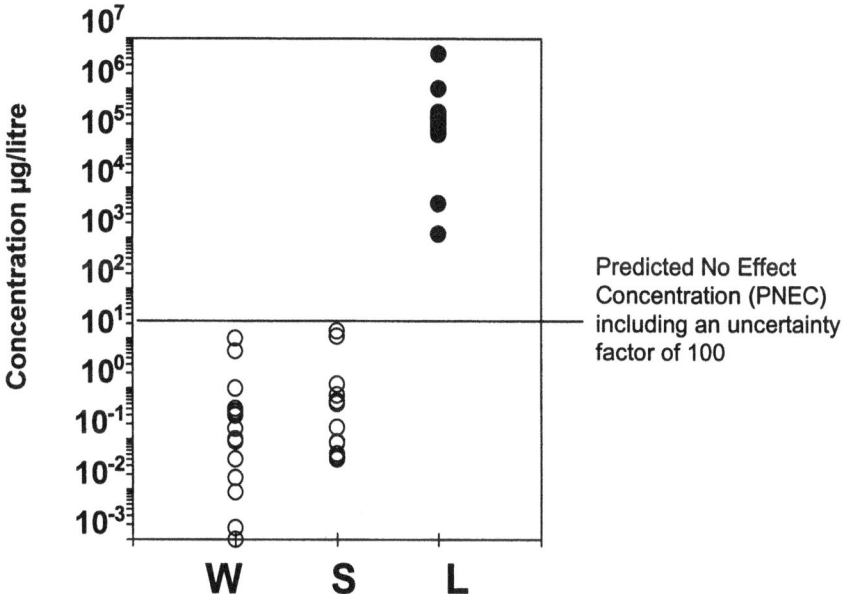

Fig. 3. Plot of measured concentrations in surface waters (W), sewage effluents (S) and reported acute toxicity values (L) for TCEP

A11. FURTHER RESEARCH

Further investigations of the mechanisms underlying the tumorigenicity of TCEP are needed.

A12. PREVIOUS EVALUATIONS BY INTERNATIONAL BODIES

The International Agency for Research on Cancer evaluated tris(2-chloroethyl) phosphate in 1989 and concluded:

a) "There is inadequate evidence for the carcinogenicity of tris(2-chloroethyl) phosphate in experimental animals.

b) No data were available from studies in humans on the carcinogenicity of tris(2-chloroethyl) phosphate.

c) Tris(2-chloroethyl) phosphate is not classifiable as to its carcinogenicity to humans" (Group 3) (IARC, 1990).

REFERENCES

Adachi K, Mitsuhashi M, & Ohkuni N (1984) Pesticides and trialkyl phosphates in tap water (Japan). Hyogo-ken Eisei Kenkyusho Kenkyu Hokoku, 19: 1–6 (Abstract).

Ahrens VD, Maylin GA, Henion JD, St. John LE Jr, & Lisk DJ (1979) Fabric release, fish toxicity and water stability of the flame retardant, Fyrol Fr-2. Bull Environ Contam Toxicol, 21 (3): 409–412.

Akzo (1995) Safety data sheet: Fyrol PCF. Amersfoort, The Netherlands, Akzo Nobel.

Akzo (1997a) Material safety data sheet: Fyrol PCF. Amersfoort, The Netherlands, Akzo Nobel.

Akzo (1997b) Material safety data sheet: Fyrol FR-2. Amersfoort, The Netherlands, Akzo Nobel.

Anderson BT (1990a) Amgard TMCP: Acute inhalation toxicity study in rats. Tranent, Scotland, Inveresk Research International (Report No. 7292).

Anderson BT (1990b) Amgard TDCP: Acute inhalation toxicity study in rats. Tranent, Scotland, Inveresk Research International (Report No. 7293).

Anon (1980) An Ames Salmonella/mammalian microsome mutagenesis assay for determination of potential mutagenecity of tris (2-chloropropyl) phosphate (Report No. 471-80).

Anon (1981a) The acute oral toxicity of tris (2-chloropropyl) phosphate Antiblaze 80 in albino rats (Report No. 2427-80).

Anon (1981b) A murine lymphoma mutagenesis assay, heterozygous at the thymidine kinase locus for the determination of the potential mutagenicity of Antiblaze 80 (Report No. 2422-80).

Aulette CS & Hogan GK (1981) A two-year oral toxicity/carcinogenicity study of Fyrol FR-2 in rats. East Millstone, New Jersey, Bio/dynamics, Inc. (Report No. 77-2016).

Barcelo D, Porte C, Cid J, & Albaigés J (1990) Determination of organophosphorus compounds in Mediterranean coastal waters and biota samples using gas chromatography with nitrogen — phosphorus and chemical — ionization mass spectrometric detection. Int J Environ Anal Chem, 38: 199–209.

Bayer AG (1986) Din safety data sheet: Disflamoll. Leverkusen, Germany, Bayer AG.

Bedient PB, Springer NK, Baca E, Bouvette TC, Hutchins SR, & Tomson MB (1983) Ground-water transport from wastewater infiltration. J Environ Eng, 109: 485–501.

Benoit FM & Lebel GL (1986) Precision and accuracy of concurrent multicomponent multiclass analysis of drinking water extracts by GC/MS. Bull Environ Contam Toxicol, 37: 686–691.

Bertoniere NR & Rowland SP (1977) Effectiveness of prepolymers from tris (1,3-dichloro-2-propyl) phosphate and polyethyleneimine as flame retardants for cotton-containing fabrics. Text Res J, 47(2): 82–86.

Brauch HJ & Kühn W (1988) Organic micropollutants in the River Rhine and in drinking water treatment (Ger.). Gas-Wasserfach Wasser/Abwasser, 129: 189–196.

Brusick DJ & Jagannath DR (1977) Sex-linked recessive lethal assay in Drosophila evaluation of Fyrol FR-2: Final report. Richmond, California, Stauffer Chemical Company, Western Research Center.

Brusick D, Matheson D, Jagannath DR, Goode S, Lebowitz H, Reed M, Roy G, & Benson S (1980) A comparison of the genotoxic properties of tris (2,3-dibromopropyl) phosphate and tris (1,3-dichloropropyl) phosphate in a battery of short-term bioassays. J Environ Pathol Toxicol, **3**: 207–226.

Bullock CH & Kamienski FX (1972) Richmond, California, Stauffer Chemical Company, Western Research Center (Report No. T-4055).

Burchill P, Herod AA, Marsh KM, & Pritchard E (1983) Gas chromatography in water analysis. II. Selective detection methods. Water Res, **17**: 1905–1916.

Burka LT, Sanders JM, Herr DW, & Matthews HB (1991) Metabolism of tris (2-chloroethyl) phosphate in rats and mice. Drug Metab Dispos, **19**(2): 443–447.

Chapman DE, Michener SR, & Powis G (1991) Metabolism of the flame retardant plasticizer tris (2-chloroethyl) phosphate by human and rat liver preparations. Fundam Appl Toxicol, **17**: 215–224.

Chemical Information Systems (1988) Information system for hazardous organics in water (ISHOW). Baltimore, Maryland, Infrared Search System (IRSS), Mass Spectral Search System (MSSS).

Cuthbert JA (1989a) Tolgard TDCP MK1: Acute oral toxicity (LD_{50}) test in rats. Musselburgh, Scotland, Inveresk Research International (Report No. 5689).

Cuthbert JA (1989b) Tolgard TDCP MK1: Acute dermal toxicity (LD_{50}) test in rats. Musselburgh, Scotland, Inveresk Research International (Report No. 5690).

Cuthbert JA (1989c) Tolgard TDCP MK1: Acute dermal irritation test in rabbits. Musselburgh, Scotland, Inveresk Research International (Report No. 5691).

Cuthbert JA (1989d) Tolgard TMCP: Acute oral toxicity (LD_{50}) test in rats. Musselburgh, Scotland, Inveresk Research International (Report No. 5694).

Cuthbert JA (1989e) Tolgard TMCP: Acute dermal irritation test in rabbits. Musselburgh, Scotland, Inveresk Research International (Report No. 5696).

Cuthbert JA (1989f) Tolgard TMCP: Acute dermal toxicity (LD_{50}) test in rats. Musselburgh, Scotland, Inveresk Research International (Report No. 5695).

Cuthbert JA & Jackson D (1990a) Tolgard TDCP MK1: Acute eye irritation test in rabbits. Tranent, Scotland, Inveresk Research International (Report No. 7200).

Cuthbert JA & Jackson D (1990b) Tolgard TMCP: Acute eye irritation test in rabbits. Tranent, Scotland, Inveresk Research International (Report No. 7202).

Draft JL (1982) Identification of aryl/alkyl phosphate residues in foods. Bull Environ Contam. Toxicol, **29**: 221–227.

ECB (1995) International uniform chemical information database (IUCLID): Data sheet on tris (2-chloro-1-methylethyl) phosphate. Ispra, Italy, European Chemical Bureau.

Eldefrawi AT, Mansour NA, Brattsten LB, Ahrens VD, & Lisk DJ (1977) Further toxicologic studies with commercial and candidate flame retardant chemicals: Part II. Bull Environ Contam Toxicol, 17(6): 720–726.

Environmental Agency Japan (1983) Environmental monitoring of chemicals: Environmental survey report of FY 1980 and 1981. Tokyo, Environmental Agency Japan, Office of Health Studies, Department of Environmental Health.

Environmental Agency Japan (1987) Chemicals in the environment: Report on environmental survey and wildlife monitoring of chemicals in FY 1984 and 1985. Tokyo, Environmental Agency Japan, Office of Health Studies, Department of Environmental Health.

Fincher KW, Guise GB, & White MA (1973) Machine-washable flame-resistant wool. Text Res J, 43(10): 623–625.

Fukushima M, Kawai S, Chikami S, & Morioka T (1986) Urban runoff as a source of selected chemicals to river waters: An observation at Isojima sampling station in the Yodo River Basin (Annual Report of the Osaka City Institute of Public Health). Health Environ Sci, 49: 11–20.

Fukushima M, Kawai S, & Yamaguchi Y (1992) Behavior of organophosphoric acid triesters in Japanese riverine and coastal environment. Water Sci Technol, 25(11): 271–278.

Galassi S (1991) Organophosphorus compounds in the River Po and in the Northern Adriatic. Toxicol Environ Chem, 31/32: 291–296.

Galassi S, Guzzella L, & Sora S (1989) Mutagenic potential of drinking waters from surface supplies in Northern Italy. Environ Toxicol Chem, 8: 109–116.

Galloway SM, Armstrong MJ, Reuben C, Colman S, Brown B, Cannon C, Bloom AD, Nakamura F, Ahmed M, Duk S, Rimpo J, Margolin BH, Resnick MA, Anderson B, & Zeiger E (1987) Chromosome aberrations and sister chromatid exchanges in Chinese hamster ovary cells: Evaluations of 108 chemicals. Environ Mol Mutagen, 10(suppl 10): 1–175.

Gardner JR (1987) Acute oral toxicity to rats of trichloropropyl phosphate. Huntingdon, England, Huntingdon Research Centre Ltd (Report No. 871285D/CLD 23/AC).

Gartrell MJ, Craun JC, Podrebarac DS, & Gunderson EL (1985a) Pesticides, selected elements and other chemicals in infant and toddler total diet samples, 1978–1979. J Assoc Off Anal Chem, 68(5): 842–861.

Gartrell MJ, Craun JC, Podrebarac DS, & Gunderson EL (1985b) Pesticides, selected elements, and other chemicals in infant and toddler total diet samples, 1979–1980. J Assoc Off Anal Chem, 68(6): 1163–1183.

Gartrell MJ, Craun JC, Podrebarac DS, & Gunderson EL (1986) Chemical contaminants monitoring: Pesticides, selected elements and other chemicals in infant and toddler total diet samples, October 1980–March 1982. J Assoc Off Anal Chem, 69(1): 123–145.

Gold MD, Blum A, & Ames BN (1978) Another flame retardant, tris (1,3-dichloro-2-propyl) phosphate, and its expected metabolites are mutagens. Science, 200(4342): 785–787.

Gordon EB (1980) Dermal toxicity of tris (2-chloropropyl) phosphate, Lot PP-28, in albino rabbits after a single exposure (revised). Princeton, New Jersey, Mobil Environmental and Health Science Laboratory (Study No. 462-80).

Gulati DK, Barnes LH, Chapin RE, & Heindel J (1991) Final report on the reproductive toxicity of tris (2-chloroethyl) phosphate: Reproduction and fertility assessment in Swiss CD-1 mice when administered via gavage. Springfield, Virginia, National Technical Information Service.

Haraguchi K, Yamashita T, & Shigemori N (1985) Sampling and analysis of phosphoric acid triesters in ambient air. Air Pollut Ind Hyg, **20** (6): 407–415.

Hardin BD (1987) A recommended protocol for the Chernoff/Kavlock preliminary developmental toxicity test and a proposed method for assigning priority scores based on results of that test. Teratog Carcinog Mutagen, **7**: 85–94.

Hardin BD, Schuler RL, Burg JR, Booth GM, Hazelden KP, Mackenzie KM, Piccirillo VJ, & Smith KN (1987) Evaluation of 60 chemicals in a preliminary developmental toxicity test. Teratog Carcinog Mutagen, **7**: 29–48.

Hattori Y, Ishitani H, Kuge Y, & Nakamoto M (1981) Environmental fate of organic phosphate esters. Suishitsu Odaku Kenkyu, **4**(3): 137–141.

Haworth S, Lawlor T, Mortelmans K, Speck W, & Zeiger E (1983) *Salmonella* mutagenicity test results for 250 chemicals. Environ Mutagen, **5**(suppl 1): 3–142.

Herr DW, Sanders JM, & Matthews HB (1991) Brain distribution and fate of tris (2-chloroethyl) phosphate in Fischer 344 rats. Drug Metab Dispos, **19**(2): 436–442.

Hoechst (1985) Wastewater - Biological investigation of Genomoll. Frankfurt-am-Main, Germany, Hoechst AG.

Hollifield HC (1979) Rapid nephelometric estimate of water solubility of highly insoluble organic chemicals of environmental interest. Bull Environ Contam Toxicol, **23**: 579–586.

Hudec T, Thean J, Kuehl D, & Dougherty RC (1981) Tris (dichloropropyl) phosphate, a mutagenic flame retardant: frequent occurrence in human seminal plasma. Science, **211**: 951–952.

Huntingdon Life Sciences Ltd (1997) Amgard TMCP 1: Acute oral toxicity to the rat. Huntingdon, England, Huntingdon Life Sciences Ltd.

Huntingdon Life Sciences Ltd (1997) Amgard TMCP 2: Acute oral toxicity to the rat. Huntingdon, England, Huntingdon Life Sciences Ltd.

IARC (1990) Some flame retardants and textile chemicals, and exposures in the textile manufacturing industry. Lyon, International Agency for Research on Cancer, pp 85–93 (IARC Monographs on the Evaluation of Carcinogenic Risks to Humans, Volume 48).

Ishidate M, Sofuni T, & Yoshikawa K (1981) Chromosomal aberration tests *in vitro* as a primary screening tool for environmental mutagens or carcinogens. Gann Monogr Cancer Res, **27**: 95–108.

Ishikawa S & Baba K (1988) Reaction of organic phosphate esters with chlorine in aqueous solution. Bull Environ Contam Toxicol, **41**(1): 143–150.

Ishikawa S, Taketomi M, & Shinohara R (1985a) Determination of trialkyl and triaryl phosphates in environmental samples. Water Res, **19**(1): 119–125.

Ishikawa S, Shigezumi K, Yasuda K, & Shigemori N (1985b) Determination of organic phosphate esters in factory effluent and domestic effluent. Suishitsu Odaku Kenkyu, **8**(8): 529–535.

Kamata E, Naito K, Nakaji Y, Ogawa Y, Suzuki S, Kaneko T, Takada K, Kurokawa Y, Tobe M, (1989) Acute and subacute toxicity studies of tris(1,3-dichloro-2-propyl) phosphate on mice. Bull Natl Inst Hyg Sci, **107**: 36–43.

KAN-DO Office and Pesticides Team (1995) Accumulated pesticide and industrial chemical findings from a ten-year study of ready-to-eat foods. J Assoc Off Anal Chem, **78**(3): 614–631.

Kawachi T, Komatsu T, & Kada T (1980) Results of recent studies on the relevance of various short-term screening tests in Japan: The predictive value of short-term screening tests in carcinogenicity evaluation. Appl Methods Oncol, **3**: 253–267.

Kawashima K, Tanaka S, Nakaura S, Nagao S, Endo T, Onoda K, Takanaka A, & Omori Y (1983a) Effect of oral administration of tris(2-chloroethyl) phosphate to pregnant rats on prenatal and postnatal developments. Bull Natl Inst Hyg Sci, **101**: 55–61.

Kawashima K, Tanaka S, Nakaura S, Nagao S, Endo T, Onoda K, Takanaka A, & Omori Y (1983b) Effect of phosphoric acid tri-esters flame retardants on the prenatal and postnatal developments of the rats. J Toxicol Sci, **8**: 339 (Abstract).

Kenmochi U, Matsunaga K, & Ishida R (1981) The effects of environmental pollutants on biological systems: 6. Organic phosphates in environments (Japan). Okayama-ken Kankyo Hoken Senta Nenpo, **5**: 167–175.

Kenmotsu K, Matsunaga K, & Ishida T (1980b) Multiresidue determination of phosphoric acid triesters in fish, sea sediment and sea water. Shokuhin Eiseigaku Zasshi, **2**(1): 18–31.

Kouri RE & Parmar AS (1977) Activity of TCPP in a test for differential inhibition of repair deficient and repair competent strains of *Escherichia coli*: repair test. Bethesda, Maryland, Microbiological Associates (Project No. T1108).

Kynoch SR & Denton SM (1990) Acute oral toxicity to rats of tris (2-chloroethyl) phosphate. Huntingdon, England, Huntingdon Research Centre Ltd (Report No. 891299D/CLD 48/AC).

LeBel GL & Williams DT (1983) Determination of organic phosphate triesters in human adipose tissue. J Assoc Off Anal Chem, **66**(1): 691–699.

LeBel GL & Williams DT (1986) Levels of triaryl/alkyl phosphates in human adipose tissue from eastern Ontario. Bull Environ Contam Toxicol, **37**: 41–46.

LeBel GL, Williams DT, & Benoit FM (1981) Gas chromatographic determination of trialkyl/aryl phosphates in drinking water, following isolation using macroreticular resin. J Assoc Off Anal Chem, **64**(4): 991–998.

LeBel GL, Williams DT, & Benoit FM (1987) Use of large volume resin cartridges for the determination of organic contaminants in drinking water derived from the Great Lakes. Adv Chem Ser, **214**: 309–325.

LeBel GL, Williams DT, & Berard D (1989) Triaryl/alkyl phosphate residues in human adipose autopsy samples from six Ontario municipalities. Bull Environ Contam Toxicol, **43**: 225–230.

Liggett MP & McRae LA (1991a) Skin irritation to the rabbit of tris (2-chloroisopropyl) phosphate. Huntingdon, England, Huntingdon Research Centre Ltd (Report No. 91198D/CLD 58/SE).

Liggett MP & McRae LA (1991b) Eye irritation to the rabbit of tris (2-chloroisopropyl) phosphate. Huntingdon, England, Huntingdon Research Centre Ltd (Report No 91209D/CLD 59/SE).

Liggett MP & McRae LA (1991c) Skin irritation to the rabbit of tris 2-chloro-ethyl phosphate. Huntingdon, England, Huntingdon Research Centre Ltd (Report No. 901196D/CLD 57/SE).

Liggett MP & McRae LA (1991d) Eye irritation to the rabbit of tris-2-chloro-ethyl phosphate. Huntingdon, England, Huntingdon Research Centre Ltd (Report No. 91210D/CLD 60/SE).

Luster MI, Dean JH, Boorman GA, Archer DL, Lauer L, Dawson LD, Moore JA, & Wilson RE (1981) The effects of orthophenylphenol, tris (2,3-dichloropropyl) phosphate and cyclophosphamide on the immune system and host susceptibility of mice following subchronic exposure. Toxicol Appl Pharmacol, **58**: 252–261.

Lynn RK, Wong K, Dickinson RG, Gerber N, & Kennish JM (1980) Diester metabolites of the flame retardant chemicals tris (1,3-dichloro-2-propyl) phosphate and tris (2,3-dibromopropyl) phosphate in the rat: Identification and quantification. Res Commun Chem Pathol Pharmacol, **28**: 351–359.

Lynn RK, Wong K, Garvie-Gould C, & Kennish JM (1981) Disposition of the flame retardant, tris(1,3-dichloro-2-propyl)phosphate in the rat. Drug Metab Dispos, 9(5): 434–441.

Matthews HB, Dixon D, Herr DW, & Tilson H (1990) Subchronic toxicity studies indicate that tris(2-chloroethyl) phosphate administration results in lesions in the rat hippocampus. Toxicol Ind Health, 6(1): 1–15.

Mehlman MA, Mackerer CR, & Schreiner A (1980) An Ames *Salmonella*/mammalian microsome mutagenesis assay for determination of potential mutagenecity of tris (2-chloropropyl). Princeton, New Jersey, Mobil Environmental and Health Science Laboratory (Study No. 471-80).

Mehlman MA & Singer EJ (1981) Four hour acute inhalation toxicity study in Sprague-Dawley rats with 2425-80. Baton Rouge, Louisiana, Gulf South Research Institute (Study No. 2425-80).

Mehlman MA & Smart CL (1981) An acute inhalation toxicity study of tris (2-chloropropyl) phosphate. East Millstone, New Jersey, Bio/dynamics, Inc. (Study No. 465-80).

Mehsl (1980) Oral LD_{50} of tris (2-chloropropyl) phosphate, Lot PP-2B, in Sprague-Dawley rats after a single administration. Princeton, New Jersey, Mobil Environmental and Health Science Laboratory (Study No. 461-80).

Meijers AP & Van Der Leer RC (1976) The occurrence of organic micropollutants in the River Rhine and the River Maas in 1974. Water Res, **10**: 597–604.

Minegishi K-I, Kurebayashi H, Seiichi N, Morimoto K, Takahashi T, & Yamaha T (1988) Comparative studies on absorption, distribution, and excretion of flame retardants halogenated alkyl phosphate in rats. Eisei Kagaku, **34**(2): 102–114.

MITI (1992) In: CITI (Japan Chemical Industry Ecology-Toxicology & Information Center) ed. Biodegradation and bioaccumulation data on existing chemicals based on the CSCL Japan. Tokyo, Ministry of International Trade and Industry.

Mobil (1985a) Static 48 hour acute toxicity of Antiblaze 80 to *Daphnia magna*. Princeton, New Jersey, Mobil Environmental and Health Science Laboratory (Unpublished report No. 50591).

Mobil (1985b) Static 48 hour acute toxicity of Antiblaze 80 to fathead minnows. Princeton, New Jersey, Mobil Environmental and Health Science Laboratory (Unpublished report No. 50593).

Mobil (1985c) Static 48 hour acute toxicity of Antiblaze 80 to bluegill sunfish. Princeton, New Jersey, Mobil Environmental and Health Science Laboratory (Unpublished report No. 50592).

Morales NM & Matthews HB (1980) In vitro binding of the flame retardant tris (2,3-dibromopropyl) phosphate and tris (1,3-dichloro-2-propyl) phosphate to macromolecules of mouse liver, kidney and muscle. Bull Environ Contam Toxicol, **25**(1): 34–38.

Morrissey RE, Schwetz BA, Lamb JC IV, Ross MD, Teague JL, & Morris RW (1988) Evaluation of rodent sperm, vaginal cytology, and reproductive organ weight data from National Toxicology Program 13-week studies. Fundam Appl Toxicol, **11**: 343–358.

Mortelmans K, Haworth S, Lawlor T, Speck W, Tainer B, & Zeiger E (1986) *Salmonella* mutagenicity tests: II. Results from the testing of 270 chemicals. Environ Mutagen, 8(suppl 7): 1–119.

Nakamura A, Tateno N, Kojima S, Kaniwa M-A, & Kawamura T (1979) The mutagenicity of halogenated alkanols and their phosphoric acid esters for *Salmonella typhimurium*. Mutat Res, **66**: 373–380.

National Medical Library (1998) Hazardous substance database. Washington, DC, National Medical Library.

Nomeir AA, Kato S, & Matthews HB (1981) The metabolism and disposition of tris (1,3-dichloro-2-propyl) phosphate (Fyrol FR-2) in the rat. Toxicol Appl Pharmacol, **57**: 401–413.

Oman C & Hynning P-A (1993) Identification of organic compounds in municipal landfill leachates. Environ Pollut, **80**: 265–271.

Parmar AS (1977) Activity of trichloropropylene phosphate in the *Salmonella*/microsomal assay for bacterial mutagenicity. Bethesda, Maryland, Microbiological Associates (Project No. T1108).

Paxéus N (1996) Organic pollutants in the effluents of large wastewater treatment plants in Sweden. Water Res, **30**(5): 1115–1122.

SafePharm (1979a) Determination of the contact sensitization potential of tris mono chloropropyl phosphate. Derby, England, SafePharm Laboratories (Experiment No. 480/911).

SafePharm (1979b) Determination of the degree of ocular irritation caused by tris mono chloropropyl phosphate. Derby, England, SafePharm Laboratories (Experiment No. 1/912).

SafePharm (1979c) Determination of the degree of primary cutaneous irritation caused by tris mono chloropropyl phosphate. Derby, England, SafePharm Laboratories (Experiment No. 119/912).

SafePharm (1993a) Acute toxicity to *Daphnia magna* (Amgard TDCP). Derby, England, SafePharm Laboratories (Unpublished report No. 071/271).

SafePharm (1993b) Acute toxicity to rainbow trout (Amgard TDCP). Derby, England, SafePharm Laboratories (Unpublished report No. 071/272).

SafePharm (1994) Assessment of the algistatic effect of Amgard TDCP. Derby, England, SafePharm Laboratories (Unpublished report No. 071/273).

SafePharm (1996a) Assessment of inherent biodegradability (Amgard TMCP). Derby, England, SafePharm Laboratories (Unpublished report No. 071/457).

SafePharm (1996b) Assessment of inherent biodegradability (Amgard TDCP). Derby, England, SafePharm Laboratories (Unpublished report No. 071/455).

SafePharm (1996c) Acute toxicity to earthworms (Amgard TMCP). Derby, England, SafePharm Laboratories (Unpublished report No. 071/458).

SafePharm (1996d) Acute toxicity to earthworms (Amgard TDCP). Derby, England, SafePharm Laboratories (Unpublished report No. 071/456).

SafePharm (undated/a) Amgard TMCP: Acute oral toxicity test in the rat. Derby, England, SafePharm Laboratories (Project No. 071/269).

SafePharm (undated/b) TCPP: *Daphnia magna* reproduction test. Derby, England, SafePharm Laboratories (Unpublished report No. 071/386).

SafePharm (undated/c) Amgard TMCP (CMW 067): Acute oral toxicity test in the rat. Derby, England, SafePharm Laboratories (Project No. 071/497).

SafePharm (undated/d) Amgard TMCP: Acute oral toxicity test in the rat. Derby, England, SafePharm Laboratories (Project No. 071/51).

SafePharm (undated/e) TCPP: Acute oral toxicity test in the rat. Derby, England, SafePharm Laboratories (Project No. 071/545).

Sala M, Gu, ZG, Moens G, & Chouroulinkov I (1982) *In vivo* and *in vitro* biological effects of the flame retardants tris(2,3-dibromopropyl) phosphate and tris(2-chloroethyl) orthophosphate. Eur J Cancer, **18**: 1337–1344.

Sasaki K, Takeda M, & Uchiyama M (1981) Toxicity absorption and elimination of phosphoric acid triesters by killifish and goldfish. Bull Environ Contam Toxicol, **27**: 775-782.

Sasaki K, Suzuki T, Takeda M, & Uchiyama M (1982) Bioconcentration and excretion of phosphoric acid triesters by killifish (*Oryzeas latipes*). Bull Environ Contam Toxicol, **28**: 752–759.

Sasaki K, Suzuki T, Takeda M, & Uchiyama M (1984) Metabolism of phosphoric acid triesters by rat liver homogenate. Bull Environ Contam Toxicol, **33**: 281–288.

Sellström U & Jansson B (1987) Mass spectrometric determination of tris (1,3-dichloro-2-propyl) phosphate (TDCP) using NCl-technique. Int J Environ Anal Chem, **29**(4): 277–287.

Shepel'Skaya NR & Dyshinevich NE (1981) [An experimental study of the gonadotoxic effect of tris(chloroethyl) phosphate.] Gig i Sanit, 6: 20–21 (in Russian with English summary).

Simmon VF, Kauhanen K, & Tardiff RG (1977) Mutagenic activity of chemicals identified in drinking water. Toxicol Environ Sci, 2: 249–258.

Smithey WR Jr (1980a) Eye irritation of tris (2-chloropropyl) phosphate, Lot PP-28, in albino rabbits after a single exposure. Princeton, New Jersey, Mobil Environmental and Health Science Laboratory (Study No. 463-80).

Smithey WR Jr (1980b) Skin irritation of tris (2-chloropropyl) phosphate, Lot PP-28, after a single application to albino rabbits. Princeton, New Jersey, Mobil Environmental and Health Science Laboratory (Sudy No. 464-80).

Smithey WR Jr (1981a) Primary eye irritant of tris (2-chloropropyl) phosphate "Antiblaze 80" in albino rabbits. Princeton, New Jersey, Mobil Environmental and Health Science Laboratory (Study No. 2423-80).

Smithey WR Jr (1981b) Primary skin irritation of tris (2-chloropropyl) phosphate "Antiblaze 80" after a single application to albino rabbits (Study 2424-80). Princeton, New Jersey, Mobil Environmental and Health Science Laboratory.

Smithey WR Jr (1981c) The acute dermal toxicity of tris (2-chloropropyl) phosphate "Antiblaze 80" in albino rabbits. Princeton, New Jersey, Mobil Environmental and Health Science Laboratory (Study No. 2426-80).

Smyth HF, Carpenter CP, & Weil CS (1951) Range-finding toxicity data: List IV. Arch Ind Hyg Occup Med, 4: 119–122.

Soderlund EJ, Dybing E, Holme JA, Hongslo JK, Rivedal E, Sanner T, & Nelson SD (1985) Comparative genotoxicity and nephrotoxicity studies of the two halogenated flame retardants tris (1,3-dichloro-2-propyl) phosphate and tris (2,3-dibromopropyl) phosphate. Acta Pharmacol Toxicol, 56: 20–29.

Sprague GL, Sandvik LL, Brookins-Hendricks MJ, & Bickford AA (1981) Neurotoxicity of two organophosphorus ester flame retardants in hens. J Toxicol Environ Health, 8: 507–518.

Stauffer (1970) Acute toxicity of Fyrol PCF. Westport, Connecticut, Stauffer Chemical Company (Report No. T1453).

Stauffer (1972) Acute toxicity of Fyrol PCF. Westport, Connecticut, Stauffer Chemical Company (Report No. T4030).

Stauffer (1978a) Mutagenicity evaluation of Fyrol PCF in the mouse lymphoma forward mutation assay. Westport, Connecticut, Stauffer Chemical Company (Report No. T6343A).

Stauffer (1978b) Evaluation of Fyrol PCF Lot 8400-3-10 in the unscheduled DNA synthesis in Human WI-38 cells assay. Westport, Connecticut, Stauffer Chemical Company (Litton Project No. 20991) (Report No. T6359).

Stauffer (1978c) Mutagenicity evaluation of Fyrol PCF in the Ames *Salmonella*/microsome plate test. Westport, Connecticut, Stauffer Chemical Company (Report No. T6361).

Stauffer (1979) Acute toxicity of Fyrol PCF - Lot No. 4800-3-10. Westport, Connecticut, Stauffer Chemical Company (Report No. T6556).

Stauffer (1980) Fyrol PCF a two-week acute dietary range finding study in male and female Charles River Sprague-Dawley derived rats. Westport, Connecticut, Stauffer Chemical Company (Report No. T10112).

Stauffer (1983a) A morbidity survey or workers employed at a Fyrol FR-2 manufacturing plant. Westport, Connecticut, Stauffer Chemical Company.

Stauffer (1983b) A mortality study of workers employed at a Fyrol FR-2 manufacturing plant. Westport, Connecticut, Stauffer Chemical Company.

Takada K, Yasuhara K, Nakaji Y, Yoshimoto H, Momma J, Kurokawa Y, Yoshitaka A, & Tobe M (1989) Carcinogenicity study of tris (2-chloroethyl) phosphate in ddY mice. J Toxicol Pathol, **2**: 213–222.

Takada K, Yoshimoto H, Yasuhara K, Momma J, Yoshitaka A, Saito M, Kurokawa Y, & Tobe M (1991) [Combined chronic toxicity/carcinogenicity test of tris (2-chloroethyl) phosphate (TCEP) applied to female mouse skin.] Bull Natl Inst Hyg Sci, **109**: 18–24 (in Japanese).

Takahashi Y & Morita M (1988) Studies on organic compounds in water. (3) Organochlorine herbicides, organophosphorus pesticides and organophosphate triesters in raw and finished water. Suishitsu Odaku Kenkyu, **11**(3): 161–168.

Tanaka S, Nakaura S, Kawashima K, Nagao S, Endo T, Onoda K, Kasuya Y, & Omori Y (1981) Effect of oral administration of tris(1,3-dichloroisopropyl)phosphate to pregnant rats on prenatal and postnatal developments. Eisei Shikenjo Hokuku, **81**: 50–55.

Thomas MB & Collier TA (1985) Tolgard T.D.C.P.LV: OECD 474 Micronucleus study in the mouse. Derby, England, SafePharm Laboratories (Experiment No. 164/8507).

Tilson HA, Veronesi B, McLamb RL, & Matthews HB (1990) Acute exposure to tris(2-chloroethyl) phosphate produces hippocampal neuronal loss and impairs learning in rats. Toxicol Appl Pharmacol, **106**: 254–269.

Ulsamer AG, Osterberg REc & McLaughlin J Jr (1980) Flame-retardant chemicals in textiles. Clin Toxicol, **17**(1): 101–131.

US EPA (1976) A study of flame retardants for textiles. Washington, DC, US Environmental Protection Agency (EPA 560/1-76-001; PB-251 44).

US EPA (1988) TCEP, TCPP, TDCPP, TCIP and TCEEP. Fed Reg, **53**(221): 46266–46273.

US NTP (1990) Toxicology and carcinogenesis studies of tris(2-chloroethyl) phosphate (CAS No. 115-96-8) in F344/N rats and B6C3F1 mice (gavage studies). Research Triangle Park, North Carolina, US Department of Health and Human Services, National Toxicology Program (TR 391; NIH Publication No. 90-2846).

Vogel EW & Nivard MJM (1993) Performance of 181 chemicals in a Drosophila assay predominantly monitoring interchromosomal mitotic recombination. Mutagenesis, **8**(1): 57-81.

Weil ED (1980) Phosphorus compounds. In: Kirk-Othmer encyclopedia of chemical technology. New York, John Wiley and Sons, vol 10, pp 488–489.

Wilczynski SL, Killinger JM, Zwicker GM, & Freudenthal RI (1983) Fyrol FR-2 fertility study in male rabbits. Toxicologist, 3(1): 22 (Abstract).

Williams DT & Lebel GL (1981) A national survey of tri (haloalkyl)-, trialkyl-, and triarylphosphates in Canadian drinking water. Bull Environ Contam Toxicol, 27(4): 450–457.

Williams DT, Nestmann ER, Lebel GL, Benoit FM, Otson R, & Lee EGH (1982) Determination of mutagenic potential and organic contaminants of Great Lakes drinking water. Chemosphere, 11(3): 263–276.

Williams GM, Mori H, & McQueen CA (1989) Structure-activity relationship in the rat hepatocyte DNA-repair test for 300 chemicals. Mutat Res, 221: 263–286.

Windholz M ed. (1983) The Merck index, 11th ed. Rahway, New Jersey, Merck and Co., Inc.

Yoshioka Y, Ose Y, & Sato T (1986) Correlation of five test methods to assess chemical toxicity and relation to physical properties. Ecotoxicol Environ Saf, 12: 15-21.

Zeiger E, Anderson B, Haworth S, Lawlor T, & Mortelmans K (1992) Salmonella mutagenicity tests: V. Results from the testing of 311 chemicals. Environ Mol Mutagen, 19(suppl 21): 2–141.

Zoeteman BCJ, Harmsen K, Linders JBHJ, Morra CFH, & Slooff W (1980) Persistent organic pollutants in river water and ground water of the Netherlands. Chemosphere, 9: 231–249.

RÉSUMÉ

1. Le phosphate de tris(1-chloro-2-propyle) (TCPP)

Le phosphate de tris(1-chloro-2-propyle) ou TCPP se présente sous la forme d'un liquide incolore. On l'utilise comme retardateur de flamme, principalement dans les mousses de polyuréthanne. Il n'est pas volatil. Sa solubilité dans l'eau est de 1,6 g/litre; il est soluble dans la plupart des solvants organiques et son coefficient de partage entre l'octanol et l'eau (log K_{ow}) est égal à 2,59.

L'analyse s'effectue par chromatographie en phase gazeuse couplée à la spectrométrie de masse. Pour doser le TCPP présent dans l'eau, on commence par le concentrer sur résine XAD puis on procède à une extraction avec divers solvants organiques.

Le TCCP est produit à partir de l'époxypropane et de l'oxychlorure de phosphore. La demande mondiale a dépassé 40 000 tonnes en 1997.

Le TCPP est difficilement biodégradé dans les inoculums de boues d'égout. Les poissons le métabolisent rapidement.

On a décelé des traces de TCPP dans des effluents industriels et domestiques, à l'exclusion des eaux superficielles. Les contrôles effectués sur des sédiments n'en n'ont pas décelé la présence. Il a été mis en évidence à l'état de traces dans des pêches et des poires crues ainsi que dans du poisson.

On ne dispose d'aucune donnée sur sa cinétique ni sur son métabolisme chez les mammifères.

La toxicité aigüe du TCPP se révèle faible à modérée après ingestion (DL_{50} pour le rat= 1017 à 4200 mg/kg de poids corporel), contact cutané (DL_{50} pour le rat et le lapin > 5000 mg/kg de poids corporel) ou inhalation (CL_{50} pour le rat > 4,6 mg/litre).

Des études sur le pouvoir irritant du TCPP pour la muqueuse oculaire et l'épiderme effectuées sur des lapins ont montré que ce composé n'est pas irritant ou tout au plus légèrement irritant. Une étude de sensibilisation cutanée a montré que le TCPP n'avait aucune action sensibilisatrice.

On n'a pas étudié la toxicité génésique et immunologique du TCPP ni sa cancérogénicité. Les résultats des études de mutagénicité *in vitro* et *in vivo,* portant sur un ensemble approprié de points d'aboutissement, indiquent que le composé n'est pas génotoxique.

La neurotoxicité retardée du TCPP a été étudiée sur des poules. L'ingestion de deux doses de composé (égales chacune à 13 320 mg/kg p.c.) à 3 semaines d'intervalle n'a pas fait apparaître de signes de neurotoxicité retardée.

Il n'existe pas d'étude consacrée aux effet du TCPP sur l'homme.

En ce qui concerne la toxicité du TCPP pour les êtres vivants dans leur milieu naturel, on a relevé, pour la CL_{50}, des valeurs allant de 3,6 à 180 mg/litre. La concentration sans effet observable pour les algues, les daphnies et les poissons est respectivement égale à 6, 32 et 9,8 mg/litre.

2.   Le phosphate de tris(1,3-dichloro-2-propyle) (TDCPP)

Le phosphate de tris(1,3-dichloro-2-propyle) ou TDCPP se présente sous la forme d'un liquide incolore de consistance visqueuse. Il est utilisé comme retardateur de flamme dans diverses mousses plastiques, résines et latex. Il n'est pas volatil. Sa solubilité dans l'eau est de 0,1 g/litre et il est soluble dans la plupart des solvants organiques. Son coefficient de partage entre l'octanol et l'eau (log K_{ow}) est de 3,8.

L'analyse s'effectue par chromatographie en phase gazeuse couplée à la spectrométrie de masse. Pour doser le TDCPP présent dans l'eau, on commence par le concentrer sur résine XAD et on procède ensuite à une extraction au moyen de divers solvants organiques.

Le TDCPP est produit à partir de l'épichlorhydrine et de l'oxychlorure de phosphore. Le produit commercial est constitué principalement de TDCPP avec des traces de phosphate de tris(2,3-dichloropropyle). La demande mondiale a été de 8000 tonnes en 1997.

Le TDCPP est difficilement biodégradé dans les inoculums de boues d'égout.

Selon certaines études, la décomposition du TDCPP est limitée dans les eaux naturelles. Les poissons le métabolisent rapidement.

La valeur du facteur de bioconcentration est faible (de 3 à 107). Sa demi-vie d'élimination est égale à 1,65 h chez les cyprinodontes.

Des traces de TDCPP ont été mises en évidence dans des effluents d'égouts, des cours d'eau, dans la mer, dans de l'eau destinée à la boisson, des sédiments et des poissons. On en a également trouvé dans certains échantillons de tissus adipeux humains.

Les études cinétiques effectuées sur des rats à l'aide de TDCPP marqué au carbone-14 montrent que le produit marqué se répartit dans l'ensemble de l'organisme après administration par voie buccale ou percutanée. Le principal métabolite du TDCPP identifié dans l'urine des rats était le phosphate de bis(1,3-dichloro-2-propyle). L'élimination du marqueur radioactif s'est effectuée principalement dans les matière fécales et les urines, une petite fraction étant également rejetée dans l'air expiré sous forme de CO_2.

La toxicité aiguë du TDCPP est faible à modérée par la voie buccale (DL_{50} chez le rat = 2830 mg/kg p.c.); elle est faible par la voie percutanée (DL_{50} par voie percutanée chez le rat >2000 mg/kg p.c.).

Lors d'une étude de 3 mois sur des souris, une exposition correspondant à une dose journalière d'environ 1800 mg/ kg p.c. a été fatale aux animaux en l'espace d'un mois. La dose sans effet observable (NOEL) était de 15,3 mg/kg p.c. par jour. La dose la plus faible provoquant un effet observable (LOEL)- en l'espèce, une augmentation du poids du foie- était de 62 mg/kg p.c. par jour.

Le pouvoir sensibilisateur du TDCPP n'a pas été étudié.

On ne peut pas dire avec certitude si le TDCPP est susceptible d'affecter la fonction de reproduction masculine car on a observé un effet toxique sur le testicule du rat mais aucun effet de ce genre sur le lapin mâle. Les éventuels effets qu'il pourrait avoir sur la fonction génitale femelle n'ont pas été étudiés.

Une étude tératologique effectuée sur des rats a montré que le TDCPP était fétotoxique par voie buccale à la dose journalière de 400 mg/kg p.c.; le composé était toxique pour les rattes gravides aux doses journalières de 100 et 400 mg/ kg p.c. Aucun signe de tératogénicité n'a été relevé.

Globalement, les données de mutagénicité montrent que le TDCPP n'est pas génotoxique *in vivo*.

Une unique étude d'alimentation portant sur deux ans a été consacrée à la cancérogénicité du TDCPP. Le composé s'est effective-ment révélé cancérogène pour le rat (augmentation de la fréquence des cancers du foie) à toutes les doses administrées (5–80 mg/kg p.c. par jour), tant chez les mâles que chez les femelles. On a également constaté la présence de tumeurs des reins, des testicules et de l'encéphale ainsi que des lésions non malignes au niveau de la moelle osseuse, de la rate, des testicules, du foie et des reins. Les lésions rénales et testiculaires étaient présentes à toutes les doses. En revanche les effets sur la moelle osseuse et la rate n'ont été étudiés que dans le groupe témoin et chez les animaux soumis aux doses les plus fortes. Dans ces conditions, il était impossible de déterminer s'il existait une relation dose-effet au niveau de ces organes.

Il semblerait également que le TDCPP ait une certaine immunotoxicité chez la souris, mais uniquement à forte dose.

On dispose des résultats d'études limitées effectuées sur l'homme à l'occasion d'expositions professionnelles au TDCPP, mais ils n'apportent pas grand chose à la connaissance du degré de sécurité qu'offre ce composé.

3. Le phosphate de tris(2-chloéthyle) (TCEP)

Le phosphate de tris(2-chloréthyle) se présente sous la forme d'un liquide jaune pâle que l'on utilise comme retardateur de flamme, surtout dans la production de résines polyesters liquides insaturées. On l'utilise aussi dans les enduits destinés à certains textiles, le PVC ainsi que les matériaux et enduits à base d'esters cellulosiques. Il n'est pas volatil et sa solubilité dans l'eau est de 8 g/litre. Il est soluble dans la plupart des solvants organiques. Son coefficient de partage entre l'octanol et l'eau (log K_{ow}) est égal à 1,7.

L'analyse s'effectue par chromatographie en phase gazeuse couplée à la spectrométrie de masse. Pour doser le TCEP présent dans l'eau, on peut commencer par le concentrer sur résine XAD ou charbon actif, puis l'extraire au moyen de divers solvants organiques.

Le TCEP est produit à partir de l'époxyéthane et de l'oxychlorure de phosphore. Depuis les années 1980, la production et l'usage de ce composé sont en déclin. En 1997, la demande mondiale de TCEP a été inférieure à 4000 tonnes.

Le TCEP n'est pas aisément biodégradable. Le facteur de bioconcentration est faible, et la demi-vie d'élimination est de 0,7 h chez les poissons.

Des traces de TCEP ont été décelées dans des cours d'eau, dans la mer, dans de l'eau destinée à la boisson, dans divers biotes (poissons et invertébrés aquatiques) ainsi que dans certaines denrées alimentaires.

Chez le rat, le TCEP administré par ingestion se répartit dans les divers organes, en particulier dans le foie et les reins, mais aussi dans l'encéphale. Chez le rat et la souris, on a relevé la présence, entre autres, des métabolites suivants: phosphate de carboxyméthyle et de bis(2-chloréthyle), hydrogénophosphate de bis(2-chloréthyle) et glucuronide du phosphate de bis(2-chloréthyl)-2-hydroxyéthyle. L'excrétion est rapide, pratiquement complète et s'effectue principalement par la voie urinaire.

La toxicité aiguë du TCEP par voie buccale est faible à modérée (DL_{50} par voie buccale = 1150 mg/kg p.c. chez le rat).

Lors d'études comportant des doses réitérées, le TCEP a provoqué des effets indésirables sur l'encéphale (lésions de l'hippocampe chez le rat), le foie et les reins. La dose sans effet observable (NOEL) était égale à 22 mg/kg p.c. par jour et la dose la plus faible produisant un effet (LOEL), à 44 mg/kg p.c. par jour, l'effet pris en compte étant l'augmentation du poids du foie et du rein chez le rat.

Le TCEP n'est irritant ni pour la peau ni pour les yeux, mais son pouvoir sensibilisateur n'a pas été étudié.

Le TCEP n'est pas tératogène. En revanche, il a un effet négatif sur la fécondité des rats et des souris mâles.

Il n'est pas possible de se prononcer sur le pouvoir mutagène du TCEP car les épreuves *in vitro* n'ont pas donné de résultats cohérents; par ailleurs, les résultats du test des micronoyaux sur la moelle osseuse sont douteux.

Chez le rat et la souris, le TCEP provoque l'apparition de tumeurs bénignes et malignes de localisations diverses.

Une dose très élevée administrée par la voie buccale a entraîné une certaine inhibition de la cholinestérase plasmatique et de l'estérase cérébrale neuropathogénique chez la poule, sans toutefois manifester une neurotoxicité retardée. Chez le rat, une forte dose de TCEP a provoqué des convulsions, des lésions cérébrales et une diminution des performances en labyrinthe.

Pour les êtres vivants dans leur milieu naturel, on trouve des valeurs de la CL_{50} et de la CE_{50} qui vont de 90 à 5000 mg/litre.

RESUMEN

1. Tris(1-cloro-2-propil)fosfato (TCPP)

El tris(1-cloro-2-propil) fosfato (TCPP) es un líquido incoloro que se utiliza como pirorretardante, principalmente en espumas de poliuretano. No es volátil. Su solubilidad en agua es de 1,6 g/litro, es soluble en la mayor parte de los disolventes orgánicos y tiene un coeficiente de reparto octanol/agua de 2,59.

El análisis se realiza mediante cromatografía de gases/ espectrometría de masas (CG/EM). La concentración de TCPP a partir del agua antes del análisis se puede conseguir mediante el uso de resina XAD, seguido de la extracción con diversos disolventes orgánicos.

El TCPP se fabrica a partir del óxido de propileno y el oxicloruro de fósforo. La demanda anual en todo el mundo superó en 1997 las 40 000 toneladas.

El TCPP no es fácilmente degradable en inóculos de fangos cloacales. Se metaboliza rápidamente en los peces.

Se han detectado trazas de TCPP en efluentes industriales y domésticos, pero no en las aguas superficiales. No se ha observado en análisis de sedimentos. Se han encontrado trazas en melocotones crudos, peras crudas y pescado.

No se dispone de datos sobre la cinética y metabolismo del TCPP en los mamíferos.

Su toxicidad aguda es de baja a moderada por vía oral (DL_{50} en ratas = 1017–4200 mg/kg de peso corporal), cutánea (DL_{50} en ratas y conejos es > 5000 mg/kg de peso corporal) y por inhalación (DL_{50} en ratas > 4,6 mg/litro).

En estudios de irritación ocular y cutánea realizados en conejos se ha puesto de manifiesto que el TCPP tiene una capacidad irritante nula o leve. En estudios de sensibilización cutánea se ha demostrado que no tiene propiedades de sensibilización.

No se ha investigado la toxicidad reproductiva, la inmunotoxicidad y el potencial carcinogénico del TCPP. Los resultados de los estudios de mutagenicidad *in vivo* e *in vitro* realizados para investigar una gama apropiada de efectos finales indican que no es genotóxico.

Se ha investigado su potencial de neurotoxicidad retardada en las gallinas. No se encontraron pruebas de dicho efecto en un estudio realizado con dos dosis orales (de 13 230 mg/kg de peso corporal cada una) administradas a una distancia de tres semanas.

No se dispone de estudios de los efectos del TCPP en el ser humano.

Se conocen valores de toxicidad para organismos del medio ambiente, oscilando los correspondientes a la CL_{50} entre 3,6 y 180 mg/litro. Las concentraciones sin efectos observados para las algas, los dáfnidos y los peces son de 6, 32 y 9,8 mg/litro, respectivamente.

2. Tris(1,3-dicloro-2-propil)fosfato TDCPP

El Tris(1,3-dicloro-2-propil) fosfato (TDCPP) es un líquido incoloro viscoso que se utiliza como pirorretardante en diversas espumas de plástico, resinas y látex. No es volátil. Su solubilidad en agua es de 0,1 g/litro, es soluble en la mayor parte de los disolventes orgánicos y el logaritmo del coeficiente de reparto octanol/agua es de 3,8.

Se analiza mediante CG/EM. La concentración de TDCPP a partir del agua antes del análisis se puede conseguir mediante el uso de resina XAD, seguido de la extracción con diversos disolventes orgánicos.

El TDCPP se fabrica a partir de la epiclorohidrina y el oxicloruro de fósforo. El producto comercial consiste fundamentalmente en TDCPP con cantidades traza de tris(2,3-dicloropropil) fosfato. La demanda total en todo el mundo fue en 1997 de 8000 toneladas.

El TDCPP no se degrada fácilmente en inóculos de fangos cloacales.

En diversos estudios se ha puesto de manifiesto una degradación limitada del TDCPP en las aguas naturales. Los peces lo metabolizan con rapidez.

Los factores de bioconcentración son bajos (3–107). La semivida de eliminación en peces del género *Phundulus* es de 1,65 h.

Se han detectado trazas de TDCPP en aguas residuales, fluviales, marinas y potable, y en sedimentos y en los peces. Se ha encontrado asimismo en algunas muestras de tejido adiposo humano.

Los estudios cinéticos en ratas utilizando TDCPP marcado con ^{14}C mostraron que, tras la administración oral o cutánea, el marcador radiactivo se distribuía por todo el cuerpo. El metabolito principal del TDCPP identificado en la orina de ratas fue el bis(1,3-dicloro-2-propil) fosfato. La eliminación del marcador radiactivo se produjo fundamentalmente por las heces y la orina, con una pequeña cantidad en el aire expirado como CO_2.

La toxicidad aguda del TDCPP es de baja a moderada por vía oral (DL_{50} en ratas = 2830 mg/kg de peso corporal) y baja por vía cutánea (DL_{50} cutánea en ratas > 2000 mg/kg de peso corporal).

En un estudio de tres meses realizado en ratones, la exposición a unos 1800 mg/kg de peso corporal al día provocó la muerte en el plazo de un mes. La concentración sin efectos observados (NOEL) del estudio fue de 15,3 mg/kg de peso corporal al día; la concentración más baja observada (LOEL) para el aumento de peso del hígado fue de 62 mg/kg de peso corporal al día.

No se ha investigado su potencial de sensibilización.

No está claro si puede afectar a la capacidad reproductiva masculina en el ser humano, habida cuenta de su toxicidad testicular en las ratas y de la falta de efectos en el rendimiento reproductivo de los conejos machos. No se han investigado los posibles efectos en la reproducción de las hembras.

En un estudio teratológico en ratas se observó fetotoxicidad a una dosis oral de 400 mg/kg de peso corporal al día. No se observaron efectos teratogénicos.

En conjunto, los datos de mutagenicidad demuestran que el TDCPP no es genotóxico *in vivo*.

La carcinogenicidad del TDCPP se ha investigado en un estudio único de alimentación de dos años de duración. Fue carcinogénico (aumento de la frecuencia de carcinomas hepáticos) en todas las concentraciones utilizadas en las pruebas (5–80 mg/kg de peso corporal al día) en ratas tanto machos como hembras. Se detectaron asimismo tumores renales, testiculares y cerebrales. Además, se observaron efectos adversos no neoplásicos en la médula ósea, el bazo, los testículos, el hígado y el riñón. Los efectos en el riñón y los testículos aparecieron con todas las concentraciones. Los efectos en la médula ósea y el bazo sólo se evaluaron en los animales sometidos a las dosis más altas y los grupos testigo. Por consiguiente, fue imposible determinar si había una relación dosis-respuesta para estos efectos en dichos órganos.

La exposición al TDCPP produjo algunos signos de inmuno-toxicidad en ratones, pero sólo en dosis elevadas.

Se dispone de estudios humanos limitados tras la exposición ocupacional, pero añaden poca información a lo que se conoce acerca de los aspectos de la inocuidad del TDCPP.

3.   Tris(2-cloroetil) fosfato (TCEP)

El tris(2-cloroetil) fosfato (TCEP) es un líquido entre incoloro y amarillo pálido que se utiliza como pirorretardante, principalmente en la producción de resinas líquidas de poliésteres insaturados. Se usa también en formulaciones de revestimientos de refuerzo de textiles, compuestos de PVC, compuestos de ésteres de celulosa y revesti-mientos. No es volátil y su solubilidad en agua es de 8 g/litro. Es soluble en la mayor parte de los disolventes orgánicos. El logaritmo del coeficiente de reparto octanol/agua es de 1,7.

El análisis se realiza mediante CG/EM. La concentración de TCEP a partir del agua antes del análisis se puede conseguir mediante el uso de resina XAD o carbón activado, seguido de la extracción con diversos disolventes orgánicos.

El TCEP se fabrica a partir del oxicloruro de fósforo y el óxido de etileno. La producción y uso de este producto ha ido disminuyendo desde los años ochenta. La demanda anual en todo el mundo fue en 1997 inferior a 4000 toneladas.

El TCEP no es fácilmente biodegradable. Los factores de biodegradación son bajos, y la semivida de eliminación en los peces es de 0,7 h.

Se han detectado trazas de TCEP en aguas fluviales, marinas y potable, en sedimentos, en la biota (peces y moluscos) y en algunas muestras de diversos alimentos.

En las ratas, las dosis orales de TCEP se absorben y distribuyen por todo el cuerpo hasta alcanzar diversos órganos, en particular el hígado y el riñón, pero también el cerebro. Entre los metabolitos detectados en ratas y ratones figuran el bis(3-cloroetil) carboximetil fosfato; el bis(2-cloroetil) bifosfato y el bis(2-cloroetil)-2-hidroxietil fostato glucurónido. La excreción es rápida, casi completa y fundamentalmente por la orina.

El TCEP tiene una toxicidad aguda por vía oral entre baja y moderada (DL_{50} en la rata=1150 mg/kg de peso corporal).

En estudios de dosis repetidas, el TCEP produjo efectos adversos en el cerebro (lesiones del hipocampo en ratas), el hígado y los riñones. La NOEL fue de 22 mg/kg de peso corporal al día y la LOEL de 44 mg/kg de peso corporal al día para el aumento de peso del hígado y el riñón en ratas.

No es irritante de la piel ni de los ojos, pero no se han realizado pruebas para estudiar una posible sensibilización.

El TCEP no es teratogénico. Afecta negativamente a la fecundidad de ratas y ratones machos.

No se pueden sacar conclusiones acerca de la mutagenicidad del TCEP, puesto que los resultados de las pruebas *in vitro* no fueron uniformes y una prueba del micronúcleo de médula ósea *in vivo* dio resultados equívocos.

El TCEP provoca tumores benignos y malignos en diversos puntos de los órganos de las ratas y los ratones.

Una dosis oral muy alta de TCEP provocó una cierta inhibición de la colinesterasa del plasma y neuropatía cerebral a través de la esterasa en las gallinas, pero no produjo neurotoxicidad retardada. En ratas, una dosis elevada de TCEP causó convulsiones, lesiones cerebrales y alteraciones del comportamiento en un laberinto de agua.

Los valores de la CL_{50}/CE_{50} para organismos del medio ambiente oscilan entre 90 y 5000 mg/litro.